MW00880219

ASSUME THE POSITION:

Memoirs of an Obstetrician Gynecologist

Richard Houck MD

Text copyright 2015 Richard M Houck

All Rights Reserved

Inquiries to rhouck@alumni.princeton.edu

ISBN -13 978-1507661178

ISBN 10 1507661177

Dedication

To my wife: she has willingly assumed the position of friend, lover, supporter, and life long partner. I would not be who I was, who I have become, and who I will be without her at my side.

Cover Art, original watercolor, by Julie Houck

Houck

Table of Contents

Chapter 1   Africa

Recently retired after four years of college, eight years of medical training and twenty years of active clinical practice, and given the unsolicited challenge of 'change your life or change your wife' with no clear path ahead, the future was uncertain other than I chose to change my life and not my wife. The crush of paper work, malpractice worries, unruly partners, a wife unhappy with but protective of me, managed care everywhere, increasing government interference in the practice of medicine, 80 employees, a Women's Health Research organization, and an acquired occupational sleep disorder, I decided to offer myself up for volunteer work in medicine and go back to my medical roots- just caring for women - no hassles and no remuneration. Medicine as it should be: "The sick, the injured and the insane", as Benjamin Franklin stated it in 1751 when laying the cornerstone at the Nation's first hospital, Pennsylvania Hospital, where I received my training. Some might have called me the insane in this scenario for leaving it all behind at the age of 50, but so be it. It was time for me to move on and seek other challenges.

Telluride, Colorado, located in the beautiful San Juan mountain range in the Southwestern corner of Colorado, is the county seat of San

Miguel County, the most rural and least densely populated corner of the State.

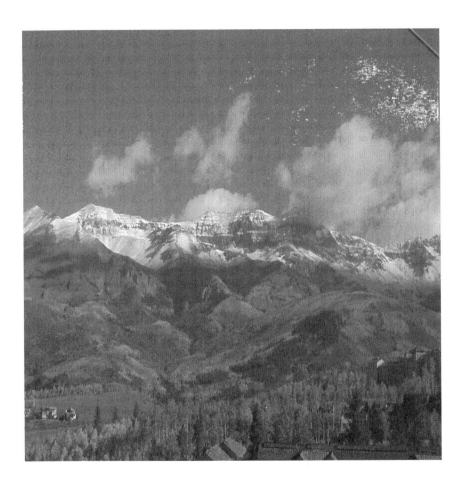

We had recently moved here after retiring from actively stewarding several thousand newborns into the Phoenix, Arizona desert. There are no traffic lights in the County. The town is located at 8500 feet above sea level and entered through the Valley Floor, home to majestic elk herds, grazing deer, foraging coyotes scouring the mounds of prairie dogs peering out of their homes on some of the most valued land in the State, occasional bears, and all surrounded by 14er's, as the 14000 foot peaks ringing the area are called.

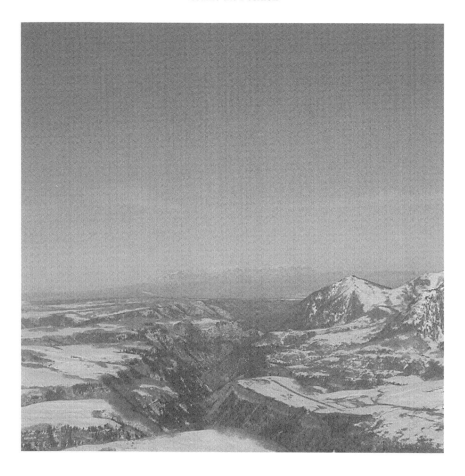

(The view from 'See Forever' ski run to the LaSalle Mountain range in Utah and over the Telluride Airport.)

Located in a box canyon, there is only one way in to the mines at the base of the mountain, then turn around and back out the other way. The fall Aspen trees were spectacular in their color and vibrancy.

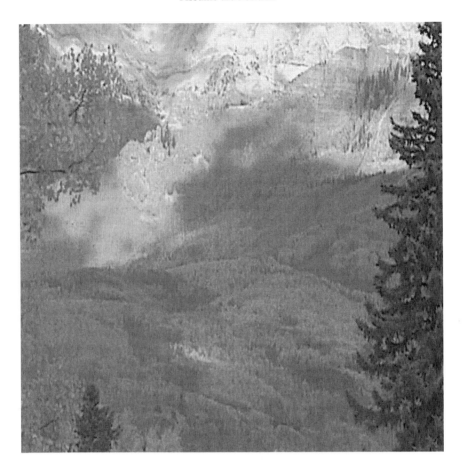

Ski slopes such as the Plunge drop right into downtown Telluride. Sure, one can drive a jeep up and over a narrow boulder strewn mountain pass once navigated only by mules, to Ouray, a 15-mile drive that takes three hours and risks life and limb. One really needs considerable off road

driving skill and nerves of steel to undertake this
venture that I would undertake when in the right
frame of mind. Every year there were deaths and
near deaths on this wondrous jeep trail through
colorful high alpine summer wildflower fields of
pink Penstemons, mauve Columbines, variegated
Indian Paint Brush, purple Lupines, and Blue
bells. There were old abandoned gold, silver and
tellurium mines high above tree line, accessible
only by the hardiest of miners with their pick
axes. The road was only passable for a few of the
summer months due to heavy snow depths.
Hardy souls used to live up there in what is a
small ghost town now, called Tomboy, during the
active mining days.

So how did I find my way to Africa to care for
women from here? There were no road signs
anywhere. Every path I had taken to this point in
my life, including the hiking trail up from
downtown Telluride, past the cool refreshing
mist of Bridal Veil falls, along one of the most
difficult jeep trails in the country, Black Bear pass,

then up the side of glorious Ajax mountain at the end of the Valley to stand on its 14000 foot peak and look down one mile onto the Valley floor that housed Telluride, was more or less well defined for me. I had made my choices deliberately and pursued them endlessly for three decades. After taking in the gorgeous scenery, the still of the green Valley far below, the coolness of what air there was at that altitude, and Ingraham falls plunging onto the carpeted Valley Floor, it was obvious to me that the path down then forward was a path not so clear. I was not sure where I was going, or what life had in store. I felt like my two miniature Schnauzers, Rosie and Lucy, who had accompanied us on this hike, darting right and left from the trail, exhausted and aimlessly pursuing the scent of Marmots yet never finding what they were looking for, outsmarted by the shrill warning sound of the sentry 'whistle pig', as they are called. The poor girls smiled at me with delight when they caught up with us and sought praise for their efforts.

Everything I had accomplished at this point in life had been a goal for me that I pursued day in and day out. I was most fortunate that I had accomplished what I had in life. But things were about to change now. It was just that I didn't know anymore what the future would bring. I was going to create a new life for myself, start over again, and see where it led me. There was a certain amount of fear and apprehension about this path into the unknown.

Making the decision to volunteer medical services is one thing, something I had often considered but never had the time to explore and accomplish. But how was I to begin? The Internet is a wonderful tool for researching this kind of thing. Dozens of organizations are out there that are happy to have people like me volunteer. I researched them all and considered them all, including Doctors without Borders. Being in the crosshairs of someone's rifle in a war zone didn't particularly appeal to me. I reasoned that if I was shot I wouldn't be much good to anyone. There are loads of faith-based organizations. As a Jew, one popped out at me from my computer screen called American Jewish World Service, AJWS. I called and began the application process. There was no discussion of where I would go nor was there any request on my part where to send me if accepted. I just put myself in their hands to see how it played out.

Interestingly, during the process of application and credentialing there was no discussion whatsoever of Judaism. They never asked if I was Jewish, I never told them I was, and we never met in person. I told them I would give a month and would go wherever they sent me. Their philosophy was based on what is called in the ancient Hebrew language Tikkun Olam, "Repairing the World". Give and receive; social welfare; people helping people. It was a simple philosophy that appealed to me. Their funds were from donations only. I liked what they were offering, which was a plane ticket, an introduction to a country, and an opportunity to do what I did best.

They accepted me after rounds of phone interviews, credential verification, and applications. They told me they were sending me to The Gambia. "Where?" I was somewhat embarrassed to ask. I had some travel under my belt, but I had never heard of The Gambia. Located on the Western horn of Africa, wedged between and surrounded by Senegal, it is Africa's smallest country with just over a million people. Wolof and Mandinka are the main languages, neither one of which was the least bit familiar to me. These were 'clicking' languages, a most unusual sound made by clicking the tongue against the palate while speaking. 95% of the people in the country are Muslim, the rest Christian. There were few white people, and certainly no Jews. There is one city, Banjul, the capital, and within the city one public hospital and one non-governmental organization, an NGO called BAFROW, the Barkus Foundation for Research on Women. AJWS gave strong financial support to BAFROW. Why? It was a good thing to do, that's all. It was about economic empowerment of women. Judaism really had nothing to do with it other than Jews doing the right thing for other people, in this case Muslim people. So right before I said yes to going, I had to ask what the deal was with religion. They had never asked me, nor me them, what role religion was to play in this month-long adventure for me. Their response was: '"That is what we liked about you. It is up to you!" So I was hooked. I chose to have religion play no role in this venture and it didn't, other than to reaffirm my commitment to my own religious beliefs.

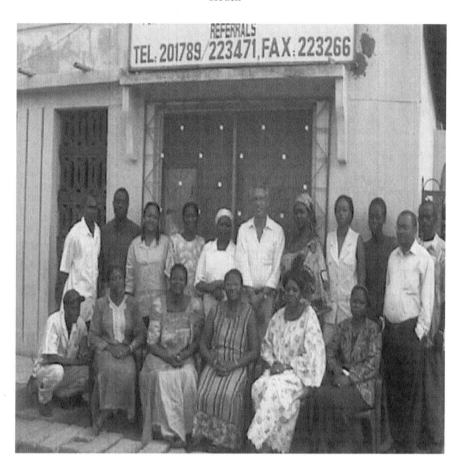

(The men and women of BAFROW, the Gambia, with me second row center.)

I learned a lot about the Gambia before going. The Gambia River goes from the Atlantic Ocean and flows in both directions several hundred miles admixing salt and fresh water. It was the lifeblood of the country. The highest elevation point in this perfectly flat country is 300 feet above sea level. There are over 500 species of birds, the main draw for white tourists. Slave trade was huge in prior centuries. Peanut farming and rice were the main crops along with cashew trees. I had never seen a Cashew tree, but I sure did like cashews. At one time Portugal had colonized the country so there was some European influence in Banjul and some admixture of Portuguese and Gambian genes. There was a King. The average man had 4 wives, permitted in Islam, and many children. HIV and female genital mutilation were both rampant.

The average annual family income was $300 per year, half of which was spent on rice for the family. So there was no hope of these people ever leaving the country, much less the continent. It was a relatively safe country. Safe, that is, if one weren't concerned about Malaria which everyone who lived there had the misfortune of experiencing multiple times. Many died from it. I learned about Lariam, a medication that I chose to take so that I could avoid Malaria since it wasn't possible to avoid the mosquitos. I was a magnet for them; they had a love affair with me.

As a country the Gambia had perhaps the world's worst statistics for both maternal obstetrical deaths and infant mortality and morbidity. There were no Board Certified American Obstetrician and Gynecologists in the country. Almost all the women had been subjected to female genital circumcision (mutilation) shortly after puberty when they were dragged into the bush and brutally mutilated by midwives with unsterile cut glass while held down by their mothers.

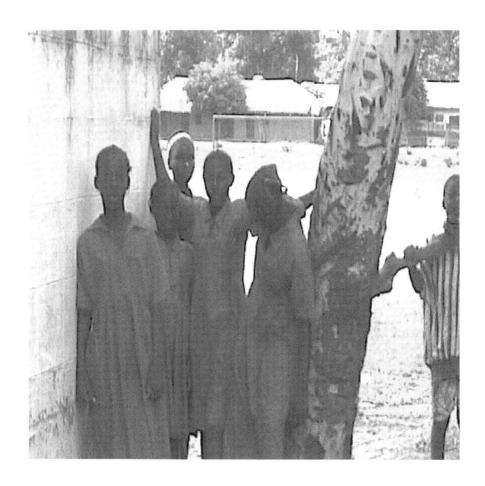

The young girls would lie in the bush without any pain medication or antibiotics until scarring began. They were brought back to civilization as women. Why did this happen? Girls were there for the pleasure of their husbands and this guaranteed that for the men. Once married a young girl would be cared for the rest of her life, so there was no escaping this horrid and brutal practice. In my prior career I had never seen the results of a genital mutilation but I read about how to surgically repair the damage since I was reasonably certain it would be staring me in the face.

There was 50 % unemployment. Most men in Banjul stood on the street corners. Most women went to work in the fields doing the hard, backbreaking work. So this was a far cry from what I was used to, that is for sure. Off I went with my huge box filled with donated materials, plastic speculums, boxes of lubrication, a microscope, and various medications I thought would be essential.

I was met at the airport in Banjul by the lovely folks from BAFROW and was introduced to the nurse who would be with me in the clinics as my interpreter. I was immediately struck by a unique smell heretofore unfamiliar to me. When asked what it was I smelled, the response was 'burning trash'. There was one clinic in the city of Banjul at the one public hospital in the country, and several in the bush run by BAFROW, all of which I would visit during the month. There was also an OB-GYN resident from Uganda working in the public hospital who would be attached to me by the hip.

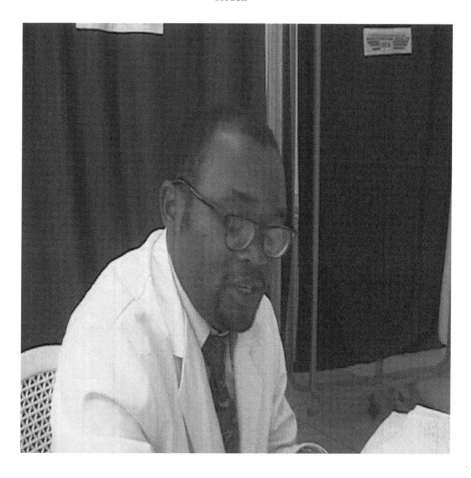

(My Resident Physician)

He was indeed a young book smart guy. But he

had no supervision and was running wild in the hospital doing the best he could to keep up with the workload. He was most eager to learn whatever he could from me during the month. And I was eager to impart as much knowledge as I could. This made us a great team.

There was one TV station in the city which blinked on and off during the day because electricity would go out on average 20 times a day. Unbeknownst to me, word got out over the TV that an American gynecologist would be in the city. The city hospital also had a unique system whereby women who had come in previously with gynecologic problems were put on a call list when help was in the country. I had no idea how they 'called' these women because there were few working phones but there they were, awaiting my arrival.

My first day at the public clinic was astounding.

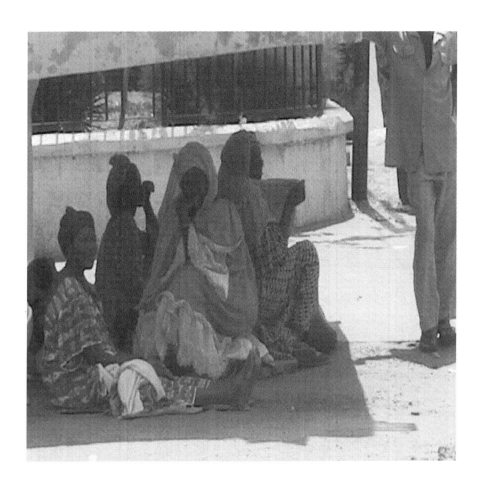

(Waiting in line in the hot morning sun.)

When I arrived at 8 in the morning, amidst

unbearable heat and humidity in July, there was a long line of women, over a hundred, hunkered down in the shade outside the hospital walls. I had no idea how long they had already been waiting. These were some of the blackest people I had ever seen. The women were most beautiful with high cheekbones, lovely white teeth, dressed in beautiful dresses made of multicolored fabrics and African patterned cloths with beautiful brightly colored headdresses. The women appeared to be wearing their Sunday finest, as we would say, that brought out the best colors and styles of all the beautiful birds in the Gambia.

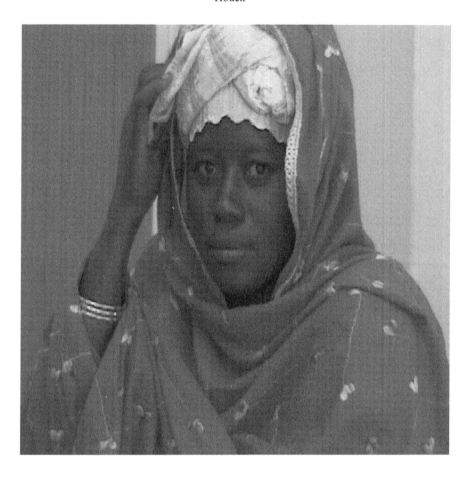

(One of many beautiful Gambian women.)

When we set up 'office' at the hospital in a

small room with an antechamber that could hold maybe 10 people, there was a mad rush to get into the antechamber and a fierce squabbling amongst the women who wanted to be the first to be seen. Our exam room had a desk, several chairs, and a gurney with one sheet on it. There were no extra sheets to be found anywhere.

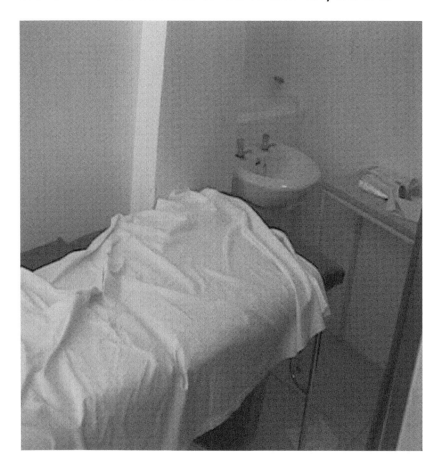

One per day would have to suffice. My specula and lubricant came in handy. I sat the resident behind the desk with me off to the side. The day began without end until well into the evening when all the women had been seen. The lines continued every day thereafter on days when surgery was not scheduled. 100 % of the women had been 'circumcised'. So to begin with they were all surgical candidates, and if all I wanted to accomplish were to correct everyone's anatomy and resultant problems there would not have been the time to do so. There were so many other surgical problems facing us that it was overwhelming, with not enough hours in the day or the month. I was distraught over how to choose who should have surgery and who not. So I made the resident make the choices. I was unwilling to decide who was more needy than the next. The only stipulation to him was that short of circumcision corrections, every case that he chose should be different from the rest. If I only had a month I felt this was the best way for him to learn. When I left he would be alone again, so he might as well see as much as he could and we should have as much surgical variety as possible. He was particularly interested in laparoscopy, a procedure that he had never seen. Laparoscopy is a highly technical procedure requiring specialized instrumentation and skills, a fiber optic light source and cables, and a myriad of unique instrumentation that had to be in perfect working order. There was one unsterile laparoscope in the hospital covered with dried blood. It had not been used in years and was far from being in perfect working order. So we spent time getting the equipment cleaned, sterilized, and in working order while instructing him and the operating room nurses how to use it.

The problems we saw on the first and every day thereafter ranged the gamut in gynecology. Infertility was huge and a major issue for the women because if they weren't able to procreate they couldn't eat. For many of these women who thought they were infertile, they weren't infertile at all. They might have had 3 or 4 children but if the other wives had produced more, in their minds by comparison they were infertile. Scarring and painful difficult labor and deliveries were the result of poor or no maternity care and mutilating female circumcisions. There were massive vesicovaginal fistulas, a complication of bad obstetrics that produced a communicating hole between the bladder and vagina so that urine constantly leaked into the vagina. Many of these women were cast out of their homes to reside in the corner of the villages since the smell was overwhelming and their husbands wouldn't come near them. Pelvic abscesses were rampant as was HIV. If a woman's husband died, his brother would become husband to them. Thus everyone was more or less having sex with everyone else with all the problems that come along with that.

Unlike medicine in the United States where prior authorization and paper work to perform surgery was required on every patient by the insurance company before taking anyone to the operating room, in The Gambia the resident just pointed and told the patient when to show up in the operating room. There were no charts or dictating machines, no insurance or related paperwork, and no malpractice worries. There was also little properly functioning equipment. In the US, when a surgical instrument or clamp malfunctioned or was bent and wouldn't work properly, it was discarded. I never gave a moment's thought when I tossed it off the operating table as to where it wound up. But now I know. They all found their way to the Gambia. When I put my hand out for an instrument it was sure to malfunction, which presented interesting challenges at the operating table.

    My first day in the operating room was an eye opener. There was a sign on the operating room door that anesthetics were in short supply and there was a visiting 'Professor' in town. All the elective surgeries other than our cases and emergencies were cancelled for the month so there would be enough anesthetic gases for our patient use.

Department of OBS & Gynae

From: Deputy Chief Medical Director

23/07/03

Date: 23rd July 2003

Subject: **CANCELLATION OF ALL ELECTIVE SURGERY TILL**
          FURTHER NOTICE

In view of the acute shortage of muscle relaxants and neastigmine, all elective cases are postponed with effect from today till further notice.

Only Emergency Surgery will be entertained by the Department of Anesthesia.

Also all Emergencies must be attended to by a Senior Anesthesia Nurse. The juniors must not be left alone to anesthetize patients.

cc.   File
      R/file

We had lined up a full day of cases. Everyone miraculously was there hours ahead of time waiting patiently for surgery. As I stood at the scrub sink with the resident for the first case of the day and went to turn on the water to begin my typical five -minute routine surgical scrub, there was no water that came out of the sink! I

looked at him and asked: "What do we do now?"
The response was that this was common. We just
put on our sterile gloves and performed the
surgery. Sterile scrubbing was out.

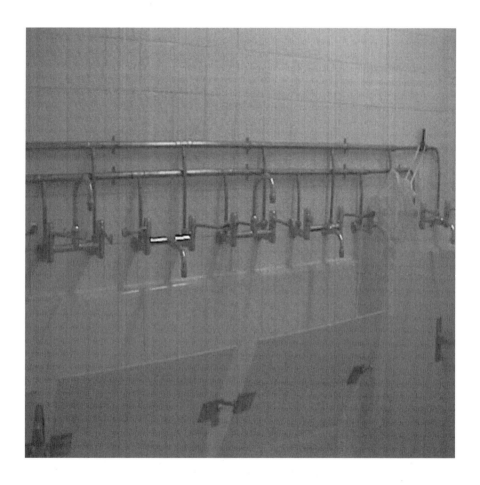

(A waterless scrub sink)

He had chosen a laparoscopy as the first case and everyone was excited to see how the equipment worked.

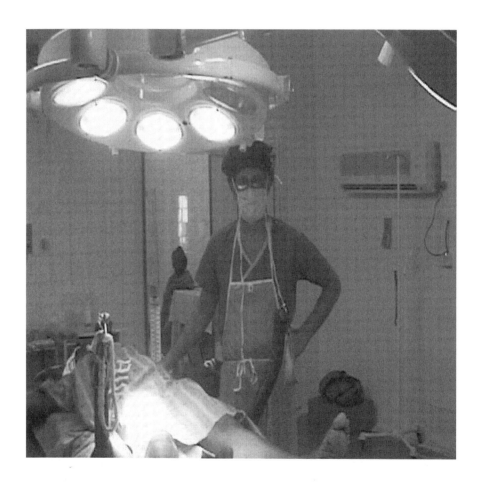

(Preparing for our first laparoscopic procedure in the Gambia.)

The operating room was windowless without air conditioning. It was boiling hot and sweat dripped. We wore heavy cloth gowns rather than the light disposable paper ones I was used to. We managed to get the laparoscope into the abdomen with the fiber optics working, identified the pathology, and were ready to begin the rest of the procedure to correct the problem when the power went out and left us in the pitch black. "What do we do now?" I asked again. This was turning into as much of a learning experience for me as it was for him. He said: "We wait, the generators will come on". Of course the anesthesia machine wouldn't work either without electricity so the nurse anesthetist began to hand bag the patient. I waited in the pitch-blackness, in the overwhelming heat, for what I considered to be an appropriate time for the electricity to come on, which it never did. When I inquired if there was an ICU and what happened to all those patients without electricity, the response was: "This is Africa, man!"

All I could think of at this point was the first and most important dictum of medicine, which is " To do no harm" to the patient. In this case we couldn't help her, but I certainly wasn't about to harm her. I took the opportunity to stress this point to the resident as we pulled the instruments out in total blackness. The first case was over! At least he had an equipment tutorial on a live patient. The rest of the cases went better that first day; an abdominal hysterectomy with removal of tubes and ovaries for a large pelvic abscess; a vaginal hysterectomy; circumcision repairs; a fistula correction. It was a full and satisfying day.

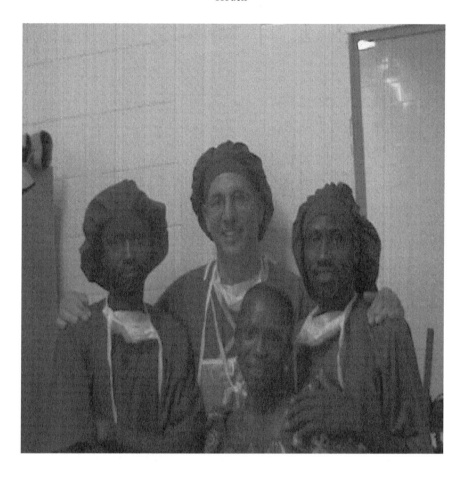

(Exhausted and exhilarated after the first
successful day of surgery.)

Upon arrival back to the clinic a phone call had come in from a local man for me. When I called him back he identified himself as my landlord. I had agreed to pay a certain amount of rent for the month I was there. Rent and food were my own expense. He asked if I was the gynecologist who had come to help the women of his country. When I said I was, he told me no rent would be necessary! Mother Nature does indeed work in mysterious ways. I felt as if someone were watching over me. Whatever fears I might have had quickly began to dissipate.

BAFROW was all about empowering women to take control of their lives.

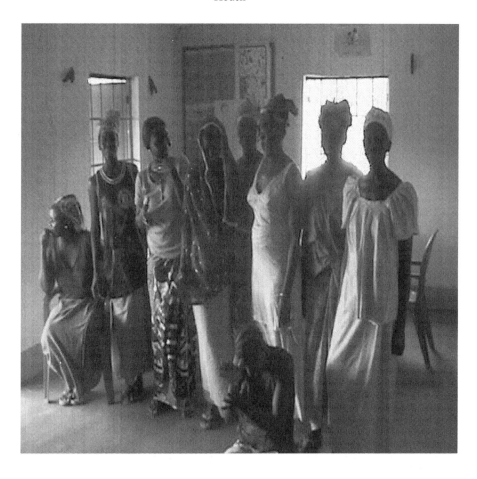

(Young women at the Bush clinic.)

Money from AJWS was used to build clinics in

the bush country; set up ways for the women to have economic empowerment for themselves in the communities; learn how to bake and sell bread and vegetables;

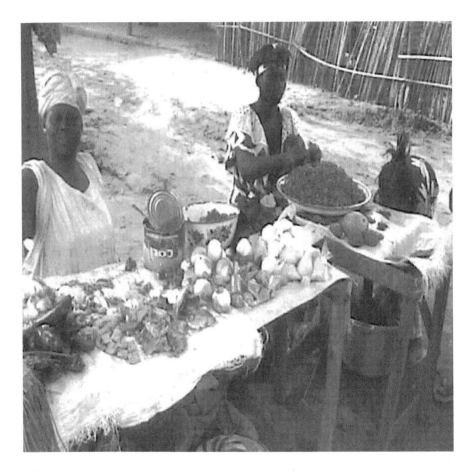

(Economic empowerment)

end female genital mutilation; build clean, new outdoor toilets; bring in running water, dig wells and in general give women a sense of self worth, dignity, and joy in their lives. The fresh bread the women made and sold outside the clinic was spectacular. I gobbled it up and bought as much as I could carry with me back to the city.

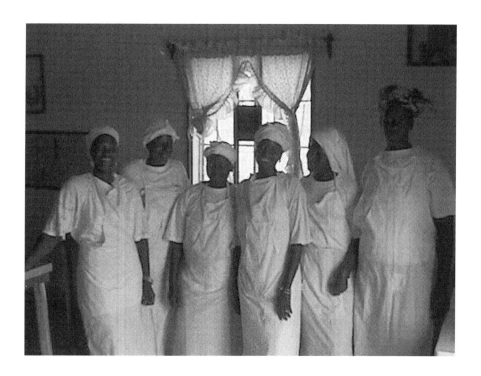

(The bakers)

Part of the arrangement with BAFROW included spending time at their clinics in the bush that required overnights in the villages. My first overnight foray into the bush country was likewise an eye opener. We drove several long, hot hours from the city along the Gambia River far inland on dirt, pothole filled roads. It was actually easier driving over the death defying, high mountain rocky roads to Ouray in Colorado than along this road.   The kids in the villages had never seen a white man before. They ran next to the van laughing, smiling, pointing and shouting 'Toubab", white man. Upon first entering the village we had to stop at the village chief's hut for a welcoming and blessing before being able to see the women of his village.

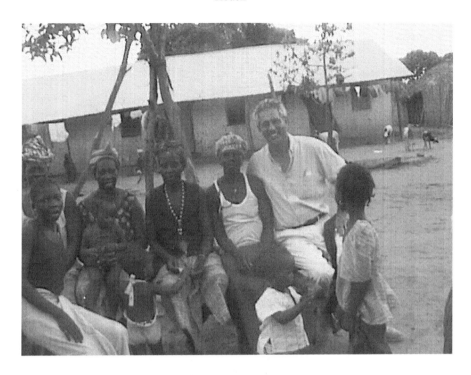

(The Village Women)

 I had been told to bring small gifts for the village chief as I did. There were midwives to be met. These women were the very same midwives who had performed the circumcisions and had now been converted by BAFROW not only to understand the harm being done but also to stop performing the procedure.

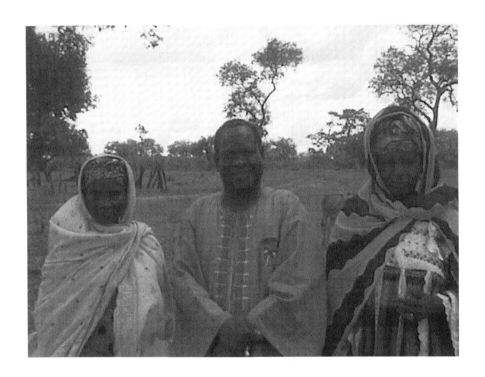

(Two former 'midwives' recently converted by BAFROW from doing female circumcisions)

Perhaps more than anything, this one act on the part of BAFROW made its very existence worthwhile. It was a slow and difficult process, however, since it was never easy to make a cultural sea change like this.

I paid visits to the local village school.

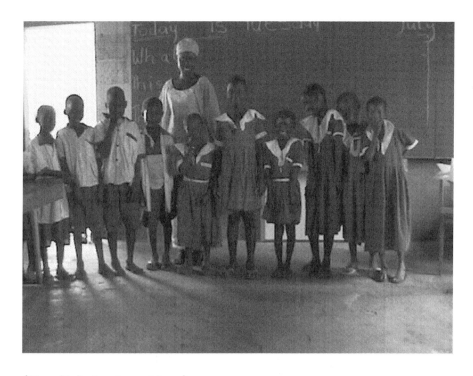

(English instruction)

The kids were absolutely wonderful, delightful and respectful, full of life and laughter as all kids are.

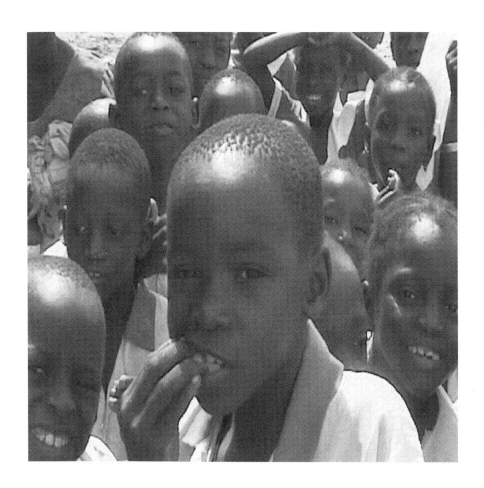

Some of the kids were mothers themselves.

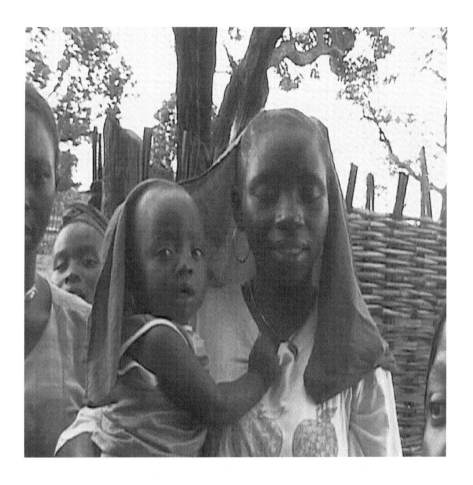

(Children having children in the Gambia.)

They were being taught ABC's so I was able to have minimal English conversation but meaningful for them.   I gave everyone the opportunity to pose questions to me through interpreters. George W Bush had just paid a visit to neighboring Senegal and promised millions in aid to Africa to fight HIV. They all wanted to know when the money was coming, as if the Brinks truck would show up tomorrow. They also asked incredibly detailed questions about how genital warts were acquired and what could be done to prevent them. This, of course, immediately told me what a major gynecologic problem it was for the villagers.

     The clinics for the women were most interesting. Invariably the first patient in line was the village chief himself. All that mattered to him was that there was a doctor in his village. He needed to be seen first despite the fact it was a woman's clinic. He had massive bunions and undiagnosed Parkinson's disease, neither one of which I could do much about other than education and a referral to the Banjul medical and surgical clinic.

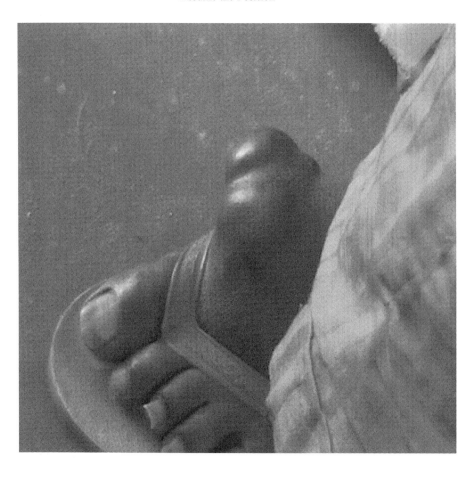

During my first clinic day four of us were wedged into one tiny overheated room; my interpreter, the patient, the largest hairy spider I

had ever seen in my life resting quietly on the
ceiling, and me.

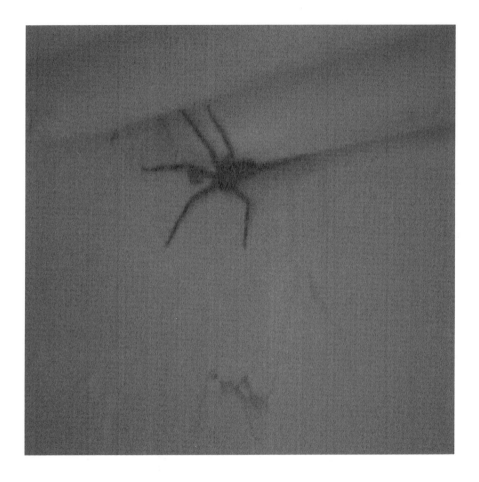

I kept my eye on it, but as the day wore on and I
became involved with patient after patient I

realized that it had disappeared when I took my eye off it. It was a bit unnerving since I had no idea where it went and the room wasn't very big.

I fully understood after being at the clinics in the Bush why obstetrical infant and maternal mortality was amongst the highest in the world. Women would labor for days often unattended or attended by untrained 'midwives', in small windowless unsterile conditions and overwhelming heat to the point of fetal death, exhaustion, dehydration, and sepsis. They were miles and hours from help. Those that were luckiest would be put on a small boat and sent down the Gambia River into Banjul, often with a dead baby inside of them for days, hemorrhaging and septic. By the time they would get to the hospital many of the women were dead or close to it. The hospital had ample antibiotics but almost no narcotic pain medication for surgical or obstetrical patients. These women often suffered alone in large wards in silence.

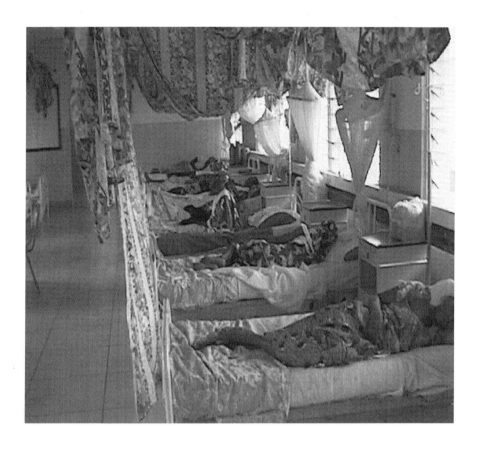

(Our postoperative ward patients covered with antibiotics but without pain medicine.)

The look of despair and death was etched in their faces. It was just a way of life. The challenges of having a healthy baby in the bush country were astounding.

I had travelled as deep into Gambia as time would allow, and it was time to turn back, to the city and eventually to home. Imagine my surprise and wonderment on my last day in the bush when at dusk I went for a stroll on the banks of the gently flowing Gambia River. It was a beautiful site despite the overwhelming heat and humidity, the amber moonlight glistening off the river, the clouds a beautiful pink and mauve, the birds chirping away endlessly discussing their day. I glanced one last time skyward to take in the moonlight again before turning back. Flying alone high in the sky was a stork, a most unusual delivery system as yet to be explored in depth by me. I had never seen one before, nor since, but it was truly a spiritual and serendipitous message for me – I took it to be a thank you from the heavens for the brief time I was allowed to spend in this beautiful country in the service of their women.

Far away from Western civilization, even far away from Banjul, the capital, these were inspiring and wonderful accomplishments in the villages as a result of the aid of BAFROW, supported by AJWS funds. I was proud to be a small part of it all and proud to be bringing health care to these women. I enjoyed the opportunity to lecture to the nursing students on various topics and to the British Medical Research Council.

UNIVERSITY OF THE GAMBIA
FACULTY OF MEDICINE AND ALLIED HEALTH SCIENCES
CLINICAL SCIENCES DIVISION

You are invited to a guest lecture

Title:
THE INFERTILE COUPLE

Speaker:
RICHARD HOUCK, M.D

Date:
WEDNESDAY, 9TH JULY 2003

Time:
3:30 PM

Venue:
SCHOOL OF NURSING AUDITORIUM
BANJUL.

You are welcome!

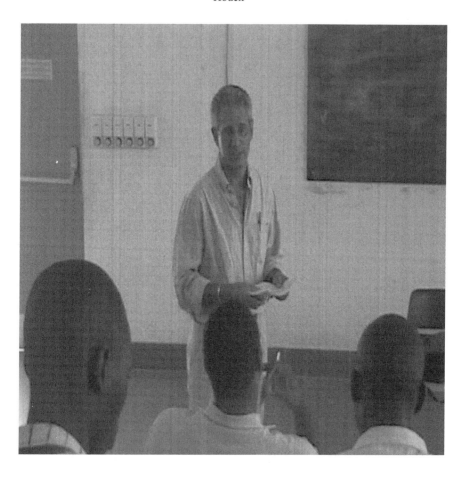

(Lecturing in the Gambia.)

I was able to establish a reliable Pap smear

system in the country and more importantly I trained the practitioners in cryosurgery, a safe, cheap and simple way to deal with abnormal precancerous conditions of the cervix and venereal warts.

I found the average Gambian outside of the hospital to be happy, smiling, and exceptionally friendly, more so than the average American. By our standards they had little money and few material possessions. Yet they smiled spontaneously, broke into song and dance for no apparent reason, and extended big open hands of greeting when passing on the street. It was a remarkably simplistic and easy way of life to get used to. I learned as much from them as they likely did from my presence.

I was asked on my return what I was most afraid of when in the Gambia. There were really only two things -mosquitoes and dogs. When in the Bush, mosquitos were rampant at sunset.

They would come out at night so sleeping under a mosquito net was critical for me as it was for everyone, though most people could not afford the few dollars that a net cost. The first night I crawled into my net and found I had company inside the net – mosquitoes. So not too much I could do about that. I placed my trust in Lariam, but it didn't make sleeping any easier. When in Banjul during the daytime I noticed packs of wild, flea-bitten and abscessed dogs roaming the streets.

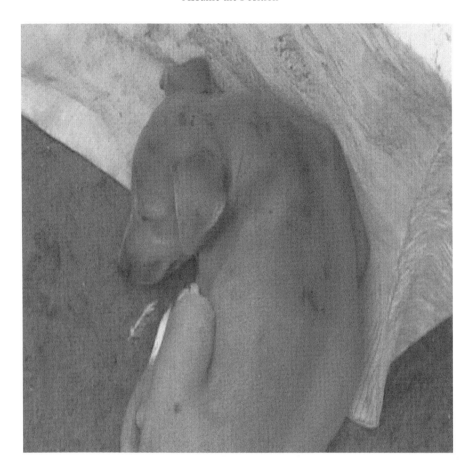

It was easy to avoid them during day time but at night, when walking around in the pitch blackness as everyone did without street lights anywhere, the dogs couldn't be seen and often were sleeping or laying in piles in the middle of the streets. I love dogs, but was deathly afraid of stepping on and into one of these piles of wild dogs at night. Everything else was easy! The folks at AJWS, and its financial supporters, are true angels!

Chapter 2 Background and Education.

A Cesarean section is the removal of a child from the uterus through an abdominal incision. The origin of the term itself has given rise to many a discussion. It has generally been asserted that Julius Caesar (100-44 B.C.) was brought into the world by this means. Likely this explanation is not correct since his mother, Julia, lived many years after her son's birth. The following view may be more plausible. In the Roman law codified by Numa Pompilius (762-715 B.C.) it was ordered that the operation should be performed upon women dying in the last few weeks of pregnancy in the hope of saving the child. In fact, the earliest Cesarean sections were usually performed on women who had already died in an attempt to save the fetus.

  Born by a Cesarean Section because my brother before me was breech, and born in the days when the dictum "once a Cesarean, always a Cesarean" held true because it was then thought that a vaginal delivery after Cesarean section was too risky for the mother due to potential scar rupture in the uterus, I was fully expected to be a girl named Ruth. For that reason I suppose I may have been a disappointment at birth. Most people who have a son would prefer their second child to be a girl. Of course I never saw it that way, but then I expect in some way it did lead to development of my gentler, softer side.

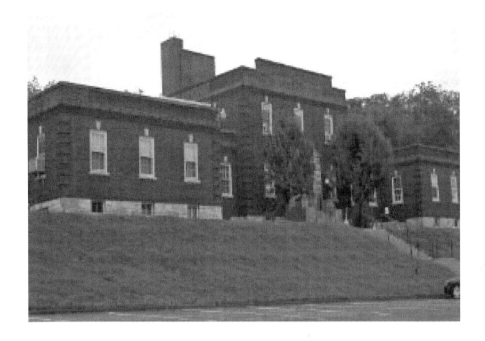

(Black's Hospital, Lewistown, Pennsylvania, where I was born in 1949)

My Dad was a small town lawyer in Lewistown, Pennsylvania, known really for nothing special other than its proximity to State College, home of Penn State.

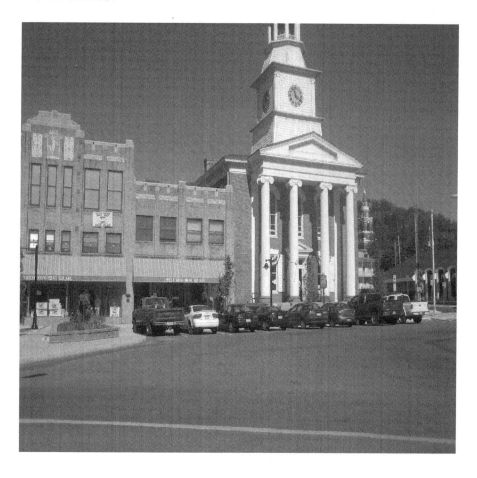

(The courthouse in Monument Square, Lewistown, Pennsylvania, with my Dad's former law office adjacent.)

He graduated from high school in an even smaller town in Central Pennsylvania, Mount Union, a brick mill town. His mother died during childbirth. Raised in a patriarchal family by their father, a shoe storeowner, Dad and his three siblings never got to know their mother. They developed a strong family support system, as is often the case in large families missing one parent, and an even stronger work ethic. He was Lithuanian by heritage, from an eastern European Jewish family, some of whom emigrated to the United States and some to South Africa. Like my grandfather, many of these immigrants were small town merchants throughout the Eastern United States. Tall and handsome, my Dad excelled in high school and graduated at the age of 16 after a successful high school basketball career. In the early part of the 20th Century one didn't need to go to college first to become a lawyer. When he graduated law school at age 19 he was too young to be admitted to the Pennsylvania Bar Association. He had little choice but then to attend college where he was again a top basketball player. His first job after law school was as a law clerk for a Federal Judge, followed by several years of law practice before he enlisted in the army during World War II in the Judge Advocate Division (JAG). He rose to the rank of Captain and became a rifle instructor, an excellent marksmen for a lefty converted to a righty, felt to be the correct thing to do in those days. He moved to my hometown of 12,000 people in Central Pennsylvania and practiced law for the next 50 years before retiring to Arizona where he died three years later. He was a kind, ethical, gentle spirit who rarely had flashes of anger, although when they flashed it was always memorable. I once made fun of his elderly sisters, who while visiting us couldn't turn off one of the 'modern' sink faucets in the upstairs bathroom. They called for help when it was too late after the sink overflowed, dripping water onto and through the floor and ceiling into the lower level. I deserved the slap in the face that I got for making fun of them. It was an impressive sight for a young kid to finally see what angered

Dad, and even more interesting to watch how my parents seemed to suggest that it was not a big deal.

My Mom was born in the coal country of Northeast Pennsylvania, Scranton. She was raised in an orthodox Jewish matriarchal family with five siblings. Her father, who was a local constable, died when she was a young teenager. The family didn't have much money and all pulled together to help out. My Mom went to a State Teacher's College in Pennsylvania. She later joined the Women's Army Corp (WAC's) during World War II, had basic training at Fort Oglethorpe in Georgia, and worked in Washington D.C. during the war. She was from the penmanship era, often writing long, beautiful letters to family in her very distinct handwriting. Although considered the Belle of the Ball, and a prized catch, Mom was 'picky' when it came to men. She held out for years until the right one came along. My parents met through a mutual friend just at the end of World War II while both were still in the Army, then married shortly thereafter at the ages of 37 and 35. My brother was born one year later, a breech, delivered by Cesarean section, and I arrived 21 months after.

For Mom, loyalty and stubbornness were close cousins, usually but not always ending up in a positive way. When Mom was on your side, she remained a loyal friend forever. But cross her for whatever reason, and one might as well not exist after that. Although family loyalty was a wonderful thing to witness, and she herself never exhibited the tendency not to speak to her siblings, there was a streak in that family that at times caused siblings not to speak for years over events that were hard for a kid to understand, and frankly even harder for me as an adult to understand. Stubbornness played a huge part in almost any major decision that needed to be made, often affecting me, rightly or wrongly. If I disagreed I was always wrong. I remember an episode years later after my Dad died. Mom was in her 80's at the time, and lived near my family in Arizona. We were out for a 'country drive' on a steep, winding, narrow back road from Flagstaff to Wickenburg, Arizona on our way back to Sun City, where she lived. She was in the back seat, my wife and I in the front. All I heard was 'bitchin' about how I was speeding on the winding roads, which I was, as she was tossed from side to side in the back. It was a fun road for me to drive, always a speed demon, but not for Mom. Of course I got pulled over by a cop. As he approached the car, and before I could say a word, she said; " What's the problem, officer? My son certainly wasn't speeding." It was the only time out of many in my lifetime that I was stopped by a cop who didn't give me a ticket. I just looked at her in the rear view mirror and smiled. Her son could do no wrong at that point in life! Even though years earlier, during my college days, we didn't speak for over a year, not a word, because she didn't approve of who I was dating at the time.

Not long after that speeding episode Mom

had a severe stroke and was incapable of caring for her self, or speaking for many months. She was adamant about remaining in her home. She got her wish, but this required full time live in help. She managed to fire just about everyone that Phoenix had to offer in the way of in home care. Often I would get a call in the midst of my busy office hours from her home aide as she was on the way out the door, saying she was leaving and Mom would be alone. 'The hell with them", Mom struggled to say. It was her way of exercising what little independence, strength, and spirit she had left in her frail body. Mom knew I would find someone else. If they weren't going to be nice to her, or stole some of her possessions, she just let them go even though there was no one else to care for her. She eventually did get her voice back after months of physical and speech therapy. It was a colossal effort on her part that spoke much of her inner strength and fortitude. Before she died she apologized to me for those times when we didn't speak, and said things to me that I wished she had said years earlier but hadn't. She was most appreciative of the time, energy, love, and attention I gave to her at the end of her life, and I was forever grateful for those last few months when she struggled to speak, this time from the heart.

My brother and I were two different human beings in many respects. He clearly relished the roll of 'older brother' and held it over me whenever he could. We played together, went most places together, and fought together. For years we had an adjoining closet between our bedrooms, and he would often taunt me with repetitive phrases such as " Bones, skinny, no muscles" over and over again while I lay crying on my bed. Although not always aware of it on either of our parts, I suspect we were just two competitive kids, whether it was competing for parental favoritism, competing on the basketball court, or competing in academics. He was the trailblazer, but often chose different trails than me. As I reflect back on it now, it didn't always make it easier for me with my parents when I went off in other directions. But the competition served us both well in our lives.

   With Penn State just 30 minutes away by car, there was no conflict about college loyalties. This was truly Penn State Nittany Lion country. There was no other team even worth our loyalties. I can still picture the long line of cars snaking through town on a Saturday morning to State College for 'The Game'. I even remember going to games on Saturdays before Joe Paterno was head coach when he was an assistant under Rip Engle. So one wouldn't be surprised to know now that after all these years of loyalty to the program, how let down I was, and still am, after the recent cover-up that occurred relating to the pedophilia scandal brought down on the school by one horrendous individual.

   Summers were spent around the local amusement park and public swimming pool, and Boy Scout camp in the mountains that garnered me nature, canoeing, and swimming merit badges. There were many car trips to visit family. The highlights for me were many journeys to Atlantic City where I got salt water in my veins, sun on my skin, salt water taffy in my mouth, and the best iced tea in the world made fresh daily by my Aunt. I could play in the ocean waves for hours on end. It was here that I first developed a healthy respect for the power of Mother Nature. One day I got carried way out past where I should have been for a little kid, and struggled mightily without success against a huge rip tide current. Scared, panicked, afraid of sharks, gasping for air, heart racing, and exhaustion setting in quickly, I felt like I was well on my way to Europe and/or the bottom of the ocean. Suddenly my feet hit a sand bar. I was able to stand up, catch my breath, get hold of myself, and figure out a way to get back to the shore. Thank goodness for swimming merit badge, good fortune, and sand bars. But I learned never to challenge Mother Nature beyond its norms, a valuable lesson for a budding Obstetrician and Gynecologist.

Law seemed to be in my family genes. My father and his brother, cousins, and eventually my brother and his wife, were all lawyers. After one summer in my father's law office, it was clear to me that it was not in the cards for my future. I was bored beyond belief, and considered myself the 'black sheep' of the family, since everyone seemed to go into the Law. But that was not to be my direction. I just needed to find my own path.

I have fond memories of two family physicians both of whom cared for us in our small town. I sensed the respect and reverence that they received within the community. I of course didn't know it at the time that I too would become a physician, but in many small ways they laid the groundwork for me. I was wide eyed when I was in their office, or when they would make house calls when we were sick as kids.

There were always distinct smells that came along with the doctor, and unusual tools and instruments that fascinated me. As a young kid home from school with a high fever, I can still remember peering through my upstairs bedroom window watching the doctor get out of his car in his black three piece suit, black medical bag in hand, slowly walk up to our front door, knowing full well the routine that would follow; greetings, peering into my mouth with a tongue depressor on the tongue, feeling my neck glands, taking my temperature (often orally, though not always), then drawing up the antibiotic into the syringe and shooting it into my behind. At the time I had no idea it was chloramphenicol, a potent antibiotic born the same year as me in 1949, now no longer in use due to dangerous side affects on the bone marrow, and of course not effective against viruses anyhow. All that mattered then was getting better and back to school as quickly as possible. But that black bag and the doctor were both full of magic, as far as I was concerned.

Two years ahead of me, my brother graduated first in his high school class and was the first kid from my hometown to go to Princeton University. I was proud of him for his accomplishments. He was an avid reader of almost anything he could get his hands on and an excellent student. He was also a good basketball player known locally as 'Big Luke' named after his idol Jerry Lucas. He had long arms and legs, and sharp elbows. Over the years I learned to defend myself with my elbows, since I got a few of his in my chest and face over the years. Taller than me, he played a great forward on our high school basketball team.

Over the next two years I had a number of occasions to visit him at Princeton. It seemed like a logical place for me to seek admission as well. The school had a great reputation, a lovely campus, and it would be fun being on the same campus with him for two years. One could actually get on the train in Lewistown, as I did many times, ride four hours through central Pennsylvania, Harrisburg, the capital city, on through the suburbs of Philadelphia, then Center City Philly, North Philadelphia, Trenton, New Jersey, and disembark at Princeton Junction. It was my favorite mode of transportation. From there the 'Dinky', a two car shuttle, would ramble for the next five minutes to deposit me right in the middle of campus facing the impressive gothic designed Blair Arch. With its massive stone steps cascading downwards from the arch to other quadrangles, dorms, and the university store, its archways would often echo with the song and sounds of a Capella student singing groups. A short stroll away was the Princeton Inn with Albert Einstein's residence nearby, all surrounded by the beautiful Princeton golf course. Walkways meandered through campus to Nassau Street, the main street through Princeton, New Jersey. One wound past stately Nassau Hall, formerly the capital building of the United States in Revolutionary war days, fronted by a gorgeous quadrangle filled with ancient, tall trees with black squirrels running up and down the trunks and limbs.   The campus was impressive, idyllic and unlike any other I had seen. The buildings were huge, mostly Gothic in design, and stately architectural masterpieces.

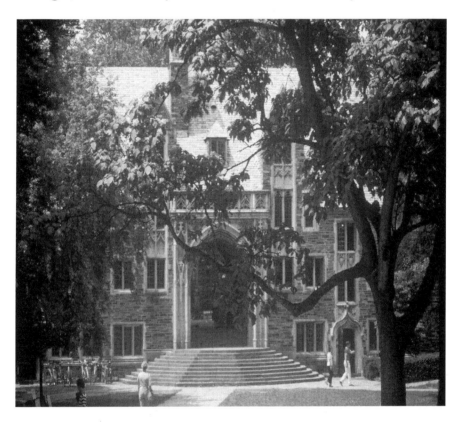

(The Princeton University campus.)

In autumn the color of the changing leaves on the magnificent trees were breathtaking. Manicured lawns were covered with red and golden brown fallen autumn leaves surrounding the Henry Moore Sculpture near the ornate University Chapel with its stained glass windows, located across the mall from the huge Firestone Library. The crisp smell of autumn was everywhere. Students in orange and black Princeton Tiger colors strolled through archways and paths scurrying from class to class. Planted by Edith Wilson, wife of former university president T. Woodrow Wilson, the amazing, formal, lovely, and ornate Prospect Gardens, located behind the president's house were most impressive. There were spectacular green clay tennis courts filled with students and faculty challenging each other. The University Tiger band played 'Old Nassau' as it marched through the campus. Crowds of alumni and students at the Saturday football games gave the campus a fall buzz of excitement and energy.

I stayed with my brother in the dorms, attended a few classes, and simply put was hooked on the place. The only challenge was to maintain the grades and scores to accomplish admission. Something like only 20% of my high school graduating class went to college, most staying in town to work in the local mill and factories. It was hardly a 'feeder' school for Princeton or any Ivy League campus. The odds of getting accepted into Princeton were pretty slim anyhow, but especially coming from our high school. So I had two more years to work at it and that is what I did. My mind was set. I wanted a good liberal arts education from the best school that would accept me. And I wanted out of Lewistown. As wonderful a community as it was in which to be raised and excel, it was too small, too isolated, and too rural for me. I knew there was a large world out there to which I hadn't yet been exposed. For me a Princeton education would be the ticket to find it.

Aside from academics, local high school sports played a big part in my life. I had a lot of mental and physical energy that needed to be expended on a daily basis. Athletics was the vehicle for me; four years of high school basketball, summer baseball leagues, and two years of tennis which was a new high school sport for me. The green clay courts at Princeton had a special appeal to me. I had never played on clay before, and I longed for the chance. I used to watch the Aussie greats Rod Laver and Ken Rosewall on TV in those long, grueling grand slam matches that went on forever in the days before tie- breakers. They were out there by themselves, with no coach to discuss how to change the momentum of a game flowing in the other direction. They often had to converse with themselves, to find new ways out of a hole, and change momentum so that things would turn in their favor. There was no one else to rely on other than one's self, which had a special appeal to me. As much as I enjoyed team sports, something about one on one head to head competition and self-reliance appealed to me.

Football was the team sport that challenged me most in high school and taught me valuable lessons for the rest of my life. Football was king where I came from in central Pennsylvania. Friday nights the stadium lights would come on, the whole town would show up for the 10 game season, good hard cider was everywhere in the stands on cool autumn evenings, and the local fans and sport pages were full of football news. There was much about football practice that I hated, and much that I loved. Two-hour practice sessions three times a day in the summer heat before the season started were grueling. If one got hurt the coaches made us 'run it off' and take laps around the field, even if the leg was dragging, the thigh bruised, or the knee swollen. Medical help was rarely accessible. Water was sprayed on the dusty field rather than in our mouths during water breaks in the midst of the summer heat. It was at times both sadistic and brutal, difficult emotions for a young adolescent to fathom, and not something any of us could ever discuss with a coach. Salt tablets were handed out before team showers because we were all in danger of depleting ourselves of electrolytes from the sweat in the hot sun with three a day practices during summer before school began.

My junior year our team went 0-9-1. One tie, and a winless season, was all we had to show for our efforts. We were the talk of the town as was our coach, a former Marine and my high school biology teacher, an all around upstanding human being. All the sweat, tears, and hard work we put in seemed wasted. My coach picked me as a captain that year. It wasn't easy being captain on a winless team. Not surprisingly, the next year someone else was chosen to be captain. I was benched for the first four games of my senior year. During one practice game I let a receiver get behind me for a long touchdown, a fatal flaw for a defensive safety. I had to earn my way back to the starting team. I unintentionally injured our best running back during practice one day, a brute of a guy with monstrous thighs. The coaches were impressed by the jarring hit I placed on him, but there were just times 'you gotta do what you gotta do' to reach a goal. After that I went on to lead our team in interceptions in the remaining six games. We won 9 games and lost one that year, the largest sports turn around ever in our neck of the woods, the heart of football in Central Pennsylvania. We won several league championships in central and western Pennsylvania. No team from my hometown has had a championship since then, almost 50 years later. Football rivalries are strange things. Mental toughness, tenacity, loss, loyalty, hard work, persistence, stubbornness, honesty, friendship, camaraderie, victory all had their roots in football for me, and to this day the lessons learned help me in my daily struggles and challenges. One of the many simple lessons I learned was never to run away from a head on challenge coming full force directly at you. Tackle it, and then move on!

When I, too, graduated as class valedictorian two years behind my brother, after four years of hard work and focus, I was asked to deliver the valedictory address at the stadium filled with parents, relatives, townsfolk, friends and neighbors. It gave me a sense of much needed comfort to do so on the field of some of my athletic endeavors. My speech focused on "The Individual". Delivered from memory because my English teacher would not permit it any other way, the speech focused on individual rights, freedoms and the lifelong pursuit of them, a theme that I took to heart for the rest of my life. Years later, every time I opened a door to an examination room in my office without knowing who or what personal situation I was going to find behind the door, I knew that I was going to respect the individual waiting for me on the exam table. That was a given.

So I followed my brother's footstep two years

later to Princeton. The unofficial motto of the University over the centuries was 'Princeton in the Nation's Service'. Past alumni who took that to heart were James Madison, Woodrow Wilson, John Kennedy (yes he started his freshman year here), Adlai Stevenson, James Baker, Laurence Rockefeller, Meg Whitman, Jeff Bezos, Bill Bradley, William Frist, and Samuel Alito, Elena Kagan and Sonia Sotomayor, three Supreme Court Justices now sitting on the "Princeton Court', not to mention Michelle Obama.

I had no idea as a freshman where I fit in this idyllic New Jersey campus. What I did know was that freshman year there was a language requirement among others. My first day in freshman German class, a language I had already studied for four years, we were all asked to stand and say something in German. I muttered through something simple about who I was and where I came from then I sat down. Next was a guy who unbeknownst to me at the time would wind up as class valedictorian four years later.

He discussed Einstein's theory of Relativity in German. I instinctively knew I was in trouble since I didn't understand it in English, and lacked the ability to express it in German. I gave my self some credit though; it was obvious I was no longer going to be at the top of my class, a good thing to know from day one.

Medicine was a thought in my head even as a freshman but in those days one had to major in the sciences to get in the hallowed doors of competitive medical schools. There were way too many other subjects that interested me to spend four years in a great liberal arts college majoring in the sciences. I suspected I could do well if I applied myself, but did not have a true intrinsic interest in pursuing science for four years to the exclusion of everything else. After an aptitude test administered at my request while in college, I remember three results: I scored equally well for professions requiring male and female traits; medicine would be a good choice for someone with those traits; I should not ever consider being an accountant since they had never seen anyone score so low in that field.

The 60's and 70's were the Vietnam era years. The campus was in turmoil and the hotbed of anti government thoughts on the one hand, with staunch defense on the part of the conservatives on campus. There was so much free speech and radicalism both on the right and left that I felt like my head was constantly swiveling. But I appreciated the accepting manner in which people were peacefully allowed to express their thoughts, no matter how extreme. It seemed like everything on TV was about war, even though no one was threatening our country. For me the wiser choice was to spend tax money to correct the social ills visible all around us if the government would just open its eyes; medical and mental health care, teen pregnancy, poor infant mortality rates, poverty, lack of higher education and lack of food for many, improvement of aging infrastructure, entitlements for the aging, and social welfare programs. War made no sense to me, nor did arms peddling and war profiteering that enriched the few and powerful.

The nation's military draft lottery system was initiated during my college years because the military couldn't get enough bodies to enlist to replace the body bags filled with dead and injured coming home on a daily basis. Perhaps one of my happiest days was when I won the only lottery in my life that was important to win, my birthday date being drawn out of the hat as number 296. It appeared the military only needed to get into the 250's to fill the body quota to fight an unpopular war. While some friends were drafted from college, others went to Canada. It was an unsettling time in the country and for me. For me, all this turmoil boiled down to what I saw I could do as an individual to affect as many lives as I could in a positive way that would make me feel good about myself and others. Medicine encompassed what I was good at academically, but more importantly I felt an emotional attachment. It was pretty simple. Helping others help themselves by providing people with the best possible healthcare, then sending them into the world to do their own thing; for me this was rewarding and a noble goal in life. It was clear to me that without one's health, it was impossible to achieve or function at home, school, the workplace, in the family, or in society. I studied all the prerequisites needed to apply to medical school: calculus, biology, general and organic chemistry, physics. Unlike my classmates I refused to major in the sciences. I reasoned that I had plenty of time in medical school for those, and wanted to branch out while still in college to take advantage of all that Princeton had to offer. I chose Sociology as a major and enrolled in a special program of Science in Human Affairs, which enabled me to explore the History of Medicine, technology and medicine, among other topics. Certainly no one, least of all my medical school advisor, encouraged me on this path. I was just exercising my headstrong independence. I needed first to understand what made people tick before I felt I could help them. Sociology and psychology were my vehicles for understanding the human mind and body and social structures. I studied poverty, education, sexual deviations, marriage, social psychology, the family unit, other cultures and societies with their ills and good fortunes. I read great works in the Humanities, studied English and literature, and the History of Medicine. In my mind this was the way to learn about human beings and what made us tick. The medicine would come later.

Women were complex and interesting for me, but they certainly had minimal presence on campus from Monday to Friday. Princeton was still an all male campus until my junior year when the university finally became coeducational and opened its doors to the better half of society. Long held patriarchal beliefs were changing on campus, albeit slowly and with resistance from the old guard. Weekends on campus women

appeared out of nowhere like manna from
heaven. There were still 'parietal hours' on
campus, which meant women had to be out of
the dorms by midnight, kind of an arbitrary hour
since if one were going to do anything 'illicit' it
certainly could happen before midnight. One
night during a raging dorm fire around 2AM the
first 30 people who came out of the dorm were
women. Although chivalry wasn't dead on
campus, it was clear that parietal hours were.
The event was captured in the Daily Princetonian
on the front -page photographs.

   There were other strange 'rules' on campus.
Young men were required to wear coats and ties
to the dining halls on Sunday evenings. So we
did. But that was all we wore one Sunday
evening. Strictly speaking we complied with the
rules. Fortunately for me there were no cameras
to capture that event.   That rule, too, went by
the wayside. Humor did have its place on
campus.

In those days there had been unspoken quotas at Princeton for acceptance of Jews and blacks. With only a few other Jewish students on campus we had no place to congregate in those days. When I graduated there were 25 black students in my class of over 800 people. A point was made at our graduation ceremony to inform everyone that there were more black graduates in my graduation year than in the entire previous 225-year history of the university system. Change was slow in those days, and has now been rectified in regards to Jews, blacks, women, and all minorities. Princeton is now a better place with the changes in favor of gender and social equality.

Princeton required all of its students to write a senior thesis, one of the few undergraduate institutions in the country to have this graduation requirement. My senior thesis was entitled the "Sociological Revolution in American Medicine", a thorough and well-researched treatise on the history of Medicine and the curriculum of medical schools that had remained unchanged over the preceding 60 years. It was my thesis that the then current standard medical school curriculum was serving the needs of current society poorly by not producing the kinds of physicians that were needed to make these societal changes necessary to improve our less than stellar national health care statistics. Compared to other highly industrialized societies, by almost any criteria one viewed, our healthcare statistics were poor. I proposed changes in medical education so that our country could begin to improve its health care delivery system, produce more primary care community minded physicians and emphasize less the need for basic science researchers.

I had a thesis advisor assigned to me in the Sociology department whom I had met only once during the yearlong writing of this tome. I had two campus jobs, four tough upper level courses

each semester, each course with extensive
reading lists, examinations, small precepts or
classes with the professors, papers to write, and
sociology departmental oral examinations for
which to prepare. I just didn't have the time for
more interaction with my thesis advisor. I knew
the deadlines and the requirements of how to
have it bound and when to have it submitted. I
wasn't interested in his critique and ideas
anyhow, a poor decision on my part, but from the
eyes of a 22 year old stressed to the academic
maximum and overwhelmed, at the time it
seemed logical to me. About three weeks before
the thesis was due I got a call from my Dad. The
Dean of the College had just notified him that I
was likely not going to graduate with my class
since I had not been working on my thesis and
had not been in contact with my advisor, as far as
they knew. It seems like it would have been
easier to get in touch with me first, but then I
was in the bowels of the library for months on
end, so no one knew where I was anyhow. Then
again I also should have been in touch with my
advisor. I turned the bound thesis in on time and

received a one-letter comment from my advisor on a 12-month project, one hundred plus page paper with over 100 references. "A". Not a single other word. I deserved both the grade, and the lack of discussion. No wonder then, that all through my years of medical school I would have a recurring nightmare that I had never graduated from Princeton, only to convince myself upon awakening that since I was already in medical school it really didn't matter.

When I graduated from Princeton, my proud parents were in attendance. Both sons had graduated from Princeton, and my brother was now at Harvard Law School. My medical school applications to what were considered top schools all over the country were still pending. Ultimately I received rejection notices from every school with the exception of one which put me on a wait list, and ultimately I was rejected from there as well when no openings occurred by the start of the academic year. The common theme was that they weren't sure I could handle the science load. I only had the bare minimum college sciences and majored in Sociology and Science in Human Affairs, the very things I had effectively argued for in my thesis that I perceived were needed for the future of medicine in this country. It was a blow to my ego, and a very unsettling and emotional time. All the hard work and dreams I had for myself, and my core beliefs about medical training and medicine as a career for me, were being tested. It was the first time in my life I had doors shut in my face, and it was not a good feeling. I needed to regroup, and figure out a plan.

Dejected, I spent the summer in Philadelphia living with my girlfriend of several years. I worked at a day camp for rich kids from 'Main Line Philadelphia', as the rail system was known that snaked through the upper crust suburbs of Philadelphia. I was the Nature Man at day camp. I had fun with the kids for a few months and developed a life long love for peanut butter and jelly sandwiches, and the outdoors. We hiked, fished, boated, played games – in general, a great way to decompress before tackling life again. After a restful summer with the kids, I found a job selling insurance and worked as a room service waiter in the evenings and weekends at the Marriott Hotel Philadelphia to supplement my meager funds. My parents, from a different generation, did not approve of my living arrangements with my girlfriend, so I financed my own life at this point. They had paid for my time at Princeton, for which I was forever grateful, but I had jobs all four years while on campus because I could not ask them to finance my social life, nor did I feel like explaining to them what it was like since I knew they would not approve. Besides, I was motivated to be on my own and was exploring life as I saw fit. Not to mention the great fried shrimp they served at the Marriott restaurant, and the loads of athletes and celebrities I served in their rooms from Maury Wills of the Dodgers, to Stevie Wonder on the keyboard, and Joe Frasier shadowboxing in the mirror while I served him.

In the fall I enrolled as an undeclared major in the graduate school at Villanova University in suburban Philadelphia, by enrolling in one graduate level course in Biochemical Genetics, which although not easy I seemed to master quite well. If the medical schools weren't sure I could do well in advanced sciences because I majored in sociology, I would show them otherwise. This time I was more thoughtful and applied to every school in Pennsylvania, my home state, rather than all across the country. I was called in to Hahnemann Medical School in downtown Philadelphia for an early interview.

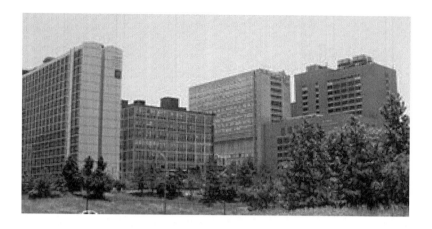

(Hahnemann Medical College and Hospital, now Drexel University School of Medicine.)

As luck would have it the professor from the admissions committee randomly chosen to interview me was a biochemical geneticist. After some brief background discussion he asked me to explain to him the difference between DNA and RNA, the intracellular basis of all biochemical genetics that makes us each unique. Fresh off my final exam in biochemical genetics, I couldn't have been better prepared. The acceptance came a few weeks later. It was an exciting time. I felt like my persistence, hard work, and commitment to a lifelong dream had been met. I withdrew all other applications in deference to those who might have been kept on a waiting list as I once was. I could 'feel' for those who might have been in the same position as I was less than one year earlier   I was going to be a doctor and would spend the next 8 years of my life in City of Brotherly love.

Hahnemann Medical College and Hospital, as it was then known, now known as Drexel University Medical School, was located on Broad and Vine streets in downtown Center City Philadelphia. It had a very strong clinical reputation, a 150 year history, and an excellent basic medical science and clinical medicine faculty. I was one of an unusual class of young and old, men and women, from all walks of life, including a nun, engineers, basic scientists, even one of our PH.D faculty members in Physiology going back to get his MD degree. My first year was immersion in all the basic medical sciences; anatomy, histology, physiology, pathology, pharmacology, biochemistry, genetics. The second year we were immediately thrown into the clinical aspects of medicine on the wards of the hospital where the underprivileged and uninsured were cared for in row after row of beds in long hospital wards. We assisted surgeons at surgeries, learned how to remain sterile when entering an operating room and how to take a medical history and perform a physical exam. Night call in the hospital was mandatory. We performed "scut" work at night, which meant starting IV's, putting in catheters, drawing blood and performing arterial sticks for blood gases.

During my subsequent clinical rotations through the medical specialties, I was most interested in Obstetrics and Gynecology and Psychiatry. I had done two clinical rotations in OB GYN, one at Reading Hospital in Reading, Pennsylvania, an affiliate of Hahnemann Hospital; the other at King's County Hospital, the county seat of Brooklyn, New York. This hospital was what was affectionately called a zoo. Babies were born in the hallways, in the elevators, all over the place and for some strange reason usually in silence. It was a cultural thing for these women many of whom were Haitian. But what a great six weeks I had. I was hooked. This was for me. Although I enjoyed immensely the intellectual challenge of psychiatry, for me it was too passive. I needed movement and activity, surgery, constant active challenges. I needed to work with my hands and fingers and move with my feet. OB GYN was all of this and more.

OB-GYN patients were for the most part young and otherwise healthy and happy. The outcomes were usually good, or at least expected to be, and not depressing as much of medicine can be. The specialty had wide variety including reproductive medicine, obstetrics, infertility, gynecology and gynecologic surgery, office care, oncology, endocrinology, contraception, and counseling. The physician was placed in the middle of people's lives. It was an exciting, emotional, and interesting time and place to be.

Aside from medicine my personal life was full, interesting, and challenging. I was on hold with long-term personal relationships at this point in my life. I simply did not have the time for a commitment to anyone other than medicine. One-night stands were preferable because they required no commitment from me, admittedly not a good way to enter any relationship with a date. It was the era pre HIV-AIDS, and after the introduction of birth control pills. Let's just say that Hahnemann Hospital in those days was much like the well-known soap opera 'Peyton Place'. Venereal disease was spreading through the medical staff, from the Chief of the Cardiac ICU, to the cardiology nursing staff, to the residents, and worked its way down to the medical students. It had no respect for the length or starch content of one's white medical coat, prestige, or stature. Gonorrhea was endemic in Philadelphia at the time. Hospitals and their medical personnel were certainly not immune, although I managed somehow to dodge the bullet.

The year of my medical school graduation, the 1976 Olympics saw Franz Klammer and his epic downhill ski race win him a gold medal at the Innsbruck Olympics. I watched this event live on TV. Little did I know I would have occasion to meet him later in life. To watch him go up against Mother Nature like that was most impressionable at that point in my life. Literally on the edge, seemingly in control and out of control at the same time was often the same thrill and feeling I had in my chosen profession, and often on a daily basis. The trick was learning how to master it and when to bail out!

Before leaving Hahnemann during my fourth year of medical school, I was asked to serve on the medical school admissions committee. I saw this as some sort of personal vindication that I had now come full circle from my college thesis and my original rejection notices from medical schools. I enjoyed reviewing applications of new potential medical students and my role in the decision making process. This was quite a turn of events five years after being rejected from medical school myself.

Choosing where to do my postgraduate training, internship and residency was a major event for a graduating medical student. There was a matching program that required applications, personal travel, interviews at the hospitals with the program directors, letters of recommendation, then finally ranking of the favorite programs by the applicants and favorite applicants by the programs. On a countrywide match day at an appointed time universal to all programs, we received an envelope with the name of the program with which we matched. We were then bound to attend this program by prior agreement, so it was a very exciting event. I matched with my first choice, Pennsylvania Hospital in Philadelphia.

They accepted only four applicants in the entering internship class for obstetrics and gynecology.

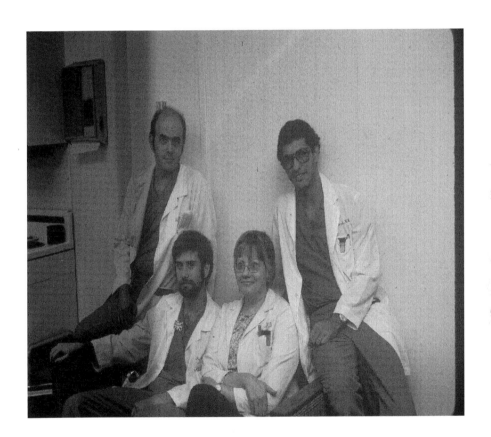

(The four exhausted interns in my first year at Pennsylvania Hospital, Philadelphia. Left to right, Steven Block, Bruce Rosen, Betty Pitcher, and myself.)

Pennsylvania Hospital, founded in 1751 by Benjamin Franklin and Dr. Thomas Bond to care for the "sick, poor and insane of Philadelphia", is located at 8th and Spruce streets, in Philadelphia, Pennsylvania. It housed the Nation's first medical library and first surgical amphitheater.

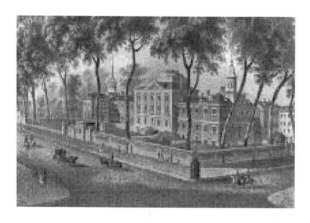

(18th Century Pennsylvania Hospital)

It currently has over 500 beds, 25,000 yearly admissions, and over 4500 births per year. Dr.

Benjamin Rush, medical researcher, social reformer, and signer of the Declaration of Independence, was on staff. The 'Lying In" or maternity hospital was started in 1803. The cornerstone of the Lying In hospital is located at 8th and Spruce Streets. Benjamin West, early American artist, donated "Christ healing the sick in the Temple", which now hangs in the historical wing of the hospital. Connecting the modern hospital with the historical wing is a long hallway covered with bronze plaques bearing the name of every intern who served the 'sick, poor and insane" of Philadelphia from 1751 until the present, including my name somewhere on those walls. Located in the old historical Society Hill section of Philadelphia, a stone's throw from the Delaware River separating Pennsylvania from New Jersey, it was a quick wintery jog in the early morning from there to Independence Hall and the Liberty Bell, down to the Delaware river, and back to the hospital, a path I often ran at 5:30 in the morning.

During my internship I spent three months in the neonatal intensive care unit (NICU) on a neonatology rotation. Neonatology at the time was a new specialty in the pediatrics realm, caring for sick babies during their first 28 days of life. The 'Father of Neonatology', one of the country's experts, was at Pennsylvania Hospital. Spending three months with him was a special experience. There were three of us in training with him during this rotation: a pediatric intern and a resident from the University of Pennsylvania, and an obstetrics intern from Pennsylvania Hospital. It was critical for us to learn how to care for sick babies. Depending where we might wind up in clinical practice, rural or otherwise, we might be the only person available to keep these young, often critically sick infants alive for an extended period of time until help could arrive. So we learned what kinds of problems put these critically ill infants in the intensive care nursery in the first place, how to intubate them, place them on respirators and make the proper respirator machine settings if they were too premature to breath on their own.

We learned how to put in umbilical lines for fluids, dosages for antibiotics and other critical medications, and how to maintain acid base balance, critical for early infant health. It was all-terrifying for me. After all I wasn't a pediatrician. The patient's couldn't communicate their medical needs. There was so much to critically assess in such a short period of time, in such a small human being. Even more terrifying was every third night on call when I was the only one in the NICU caring for up to 20 or more premature babies at times. As we were required, we attended each of the Cesarean sections as the 'pediatrician'. Although I would have preferred to be performing the delivery itself, during this three-month period I was on the receiving and not the delivering end.

One night I was called to attend what appeared to be a routine repeat Cesarean section on a mom who had arrived in active labor. Still in the "once a C section always a C section" era everything was expected to be routine with the baby, so I was expecting nothing out of the ordinary. I was handed a term baby that for some reason had awful Apgar scores, was blue with minimal shallow respirations, grunting and retracting. This was a clinic patient with no financial resources or insurance, it was past midnight, and I was it as far as pediatrics for the evening. Clinic patients were almost always entrusted to the resident house staff in training, i.e. me. I stabilized the baby, intubated and bagged it immediately, put in umbilical catheter lines, checked x-rays for line and tube placement, took it to the neonatal ICU, and waited for initial labs and blood gases to come back. When I was satisfied with the results, I called the Father of Neonatology and Chief of Service on the phone to inform him of a new admission to the NICU, apologized for waking him, gave him the details and numbers, and asked if I missed anything. He said: "Is this a fourth floor baby or a fifth floor baby?" which meant was it a 'ward' baby or a "private" baby, in his language non-pay or insurance. I responded that it was a 'fourth floor baby", meaning no insurance. He said, 'Keep up the good work and I will be in later this morning."

By the time of morning rounds, after an exhausting night with no sleep, I was so proud of the work I had done. I kept this baby alive all by myself while not only producing perfect laboratory acid base numbers but also caring for all the other neonates in the neonatal ICU. The Father of Neonatology arrived for morning rounds. When it came to this baby he took one look at it, pulled out the endotracheal tube and turned off the respirator. I was aghast. He said, "You have just saved a Mongol for the world. If he is going to live, he is going to do it on his own." I suspect he knew the infant would make it without the respirator, but I couldn't have made that judgment at that time. I had never seen a newborn Down syndrome baby before so I missed the diagnosis completely but had I made the diagnosis I would not have done anything differently. He put a name card on the baby's bassinet and called it 'baby Rick' Smith, named by him after me. Each day on rounds for the next month he would begin the presentation of baby Smith with the same comment. "Rick saved this Mongol for the world". And I did. He went home one month later.

The training program at Pennsylvania Hospital in general was excellent. Our Chief of Service, nationally renowned, had the highest standards and expected the same of each one of us. Every morning at 7:30 AM was 'Morning Report,' where all residents would gather and sit in silence as the Chief Resident of Obstetrics would discuss the statistics for births the prior day, indications for each Cesarean Section which had been performed, whether on the resident (public patients) or private (insured) attending physician service. The Chief Resident would usually come in around 6 am each day to get this information and review all the pertinent charts. Morning report was a learning experience for the whole resident staff, but no one other than the Chief Residents and the Chief of Service could speak. Among other things we would learn when

Cesarean sections should, and should not, be done. The Chief Resident on the Gynecology service would present all cases scheduled for surgery in the operating room that day. If in the opinion of the Chief of Service a case had not been evaluated or selected properly for surgery the Chief of Service would just cancel the case and send the patient back to the clinic for further evaluation, even if the patient was in the pre op holding area. Often times the surgery was cancelled for something simple like not knowing what the patient's blood count was before surgery; or an adequate medical trial of therapy hadn't been tried before surgery was entertained, or the indications for the procedure were inadequate. Peer review happened every day under the Chief's tutelage that served me well for my future endeavors. He set an example for us as to how correct medicine should be practiced. Nothing else was acceptable. It just became part of my mindset.

One night in the middle of the night I was

performing a particularly difficult forceps delivery and rotation of the fetal head while still in the birth canal. I heard someone breathing over my shoulder. I looked around and there was the Chief of service who had appeared out of nowhere, inquiring if I had met all indications for applications of the forceps, why I was using this particular forceps as opposed to another. He checked the application of the forceps to the baby's head himself, and then permitted me to continue as he watched the whole delivery, then quietly left the room, what I took to be silent approval. For me, I felt a sense of accomplishment and satisfaction that I had been silently observed, and passed with flying colors.

Multiple births were common at Pennsylvania hospital, particularly because there were world-renowned infertility specialists on staff. During one 48-hour period I had occasion as Chief resident to deliver triplets and sextuplets. The triplets were known and expected. The sextuplets were not. The mom had severe preeclampsia, a pregnancy induced syndrome that increased risk for both mother and baby, heading towards eclampsia with life threatening seizures and hypertension. We were trying to extract every hour possible out of her before delivering what we thought were her premature twins. It was a fine balance. When one baby suddenly died in utero and her blood pressure shot way up we had no choice but to proceed to immediate Cesarean Section, thinking we were going to get one dead and one living baby. Ultrasound was in its very infancy in 1977 such that the staff and residents were just learning how to use it and interpret it. Pennsylvania Hospital had one of the first Antenatal testing units and ultrasound machines. We needed it to identify how many babies we were dealing with, and whether they were alive or without heart beat. At the time of the Cesarean I put my hand in the uterus and pulled out the first baby who was alive. The second one I pulled out I of course expected to be the dead baby but it too was alive. I kept putting my hand into the uterus, pulling out living baby after living baby, while placing stat pages for more pediatricians. The first five were all alive and only the sixth was dead.

Then there was a true record multiple-birth I attended, perhaps a world record. In the 'Old Days', women in early labor would get enemas, walk, evacuate their lower bowels, and deliveries were much cleaner for everyone. Somewhere during residency in the late 1970's this process changed and/or some women refused enemas. So be it. Mother Nature is what she is. As this patient pushed with the baby's head on the perineum out from the rectum also came stool followed by a ball of white squiggly material that at first I had trouble identifying. As the ball disintegrated and began to move all over her perineum up to and over the crowning baby's head, it became obvious that these were pinworms, hundreds if not thousands of them. The Guinness Book of world records would have been proud to witness this record number of deliveries from one person at the same time. I wasn't. Watching worms crawl out of someone's rectum, over her perineum onto the baby's head, and then having to remove them was less than thrilling for me. All in a day's work, I suppose – but an experience never to forget!

Late one night a 'private' patient of one of the attending physicians was in labor. He had been there earlier to visit her and then departed for what everyone assumed would be a short rest. When it was time for her to deliver, stat overhead and beeper pages and calls to his office were unanswered. Since I was the senior resident on call that night I was expected to cover for him so I did the delivery. He never did answer or show up. Later that morning when his office opened he was found dead on his office desk. It turned out he was having sex on his desk with one of the hospital nurses and died right there on the spot. The nurse bolted and left him lying there with his pants down, so it was pretty obvious to those who found him what had happened. What a way to go! The last time I was in the lobby of this historical Women's Lying In hospital I saw his portrait on the wall next to other titans who had served the institution well over the decades. I just couldn't help thinking this story was the real reason he was being honored.

My four years of training eventually came to an end. It was true that formal education had stopped, but after becoming a member of the American College of Obstetrics and Gynecology with life long board certification, it was really illusory that education ever ended. As long as there were patients to be seen, as long as medical science progressed and changed, as long as new journals were published and read, as long as peer review remained important to me, education would never cease. It was simply a lifelong process.

With the completion of my formal training, my wife and I had decided to move to Phoenix,

Arizona where I had a nice job offer awaiting me. I was about to join two former Philadelphia physicians, one of whom also trained a few years ahead of me at Pennsylvania Hospital. While still in my residency, he had returned to Philadelphia one week to recruit a prospective partner. I subsequently went to Phoenix to visit, see the practice, and meet his partner and their families. I had always wanted to go West, but never had the courage to do so by myself. Since my wife wanted the same thing, it was an easy decision for us. We visited Arizona again together on a home hunting expedition, and for my wife to see her new community. We liked what we saw. Opportunity for both of us was everywhere. It seemed like a good place to raise a family. Phoenix was a place for the sun to shine on us! We left friends and family behind for a new beginning. My parents couldn't understand. "Where is Arizona?" they said. "And what happens when we have grandchildren?" "Fortunately there are airplanes," I explained.

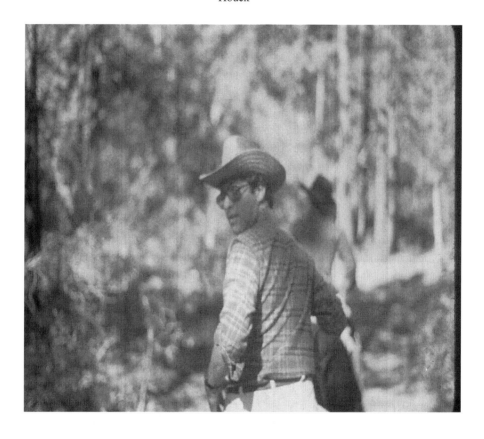

(An Arizona cowboy.)

Chapter 3   Labor and Delivery

There were many things to learn during my
internship about Labor and Delivery. One of the
things that plagued me as an intern trying to
master Obstetrics at Pennsylvania Hospital was
how long to leave a woman in labor in the labor
room before moving her to the delivery room
and table. If the timing was late she would deliver
in the unsterile labor bed; and if the timing was

early she would labor for a far longer time than desired while in the uncomfortable stirrups on the delivery room table, a situation I had difficulty mastering at first. One could read about labor and delivery all day long in the textbooks, but learning how to manage labor varied with the individual. It took years of experience, observation, and an understanding as to what was within the norms and what was outside of acceptable limits. When in doubt about these things, the best person's brain to pick was often one of the well-seasoned labor and delivery nurses. So I asked Greenie, who had been there for 37 years, for some advice.

"Doc," she said, "When they ask for the ophthalmologist (eye doctor) you know it is time to move them".

'Huh?", I muttered, scratching my head. She said it sounds like this. "AYYYY, doctor! "AYYYYYYY, doctor!"

I had been trying to figure it all out from results of my pelvic exams. She had the answer without the exams. Listen to the patient, she told me. Look at her face! Read her sense of urgency, tension, pain and emotion. Listen to the crescendo in her voice. See the furrowed brow and the sweat bead on the upper lip. Watch the little blood vessels in her face pop. A valuable lesson, indeed! I got it, and never forgot it. Why didn't they tell Greenie to just write it down in the textbook?

Most of the women for whom we cared while in Labor at Pennsylvania Hospital were young, black, poor, and often uneducated. Obviously pregnant, these women were our clinic patients, and received the best care available in Philadelphia. As residents we learned to administer our own epidurals during labor for pain relief, and although we became quite proficient at them, if the patient wasn't cooperative it was not an easy procedure. I remember well one young 13 year-old clinic patient who came into labor and delivery screaming at the top of her lungs without a support person. She was out of control, writhing in bed, on all fours at times, alternatively climbing over the bed rails and standing on the bed, refusing an examination and refusing to be touched or to even have an IV placed. No amount of calm persuasion, talking, or any sort of communication was effective. She was demanding pain medication. I did my best to explain to her that nothing was going to happen to help her unless she cooperated, we were not going to do anything to hurt her or her baby, and nothing could be done until we examined her first. She refused. There were only two or three times in my career when I raised my voice to a patient, this being the first. It only happened as a last resort when education, communication, discussion, calm persuasion, and all else failed. I closed the door to the labor room so that it was just she and I. In no uncertain terms, with a calm but raised voice, I explained to her that I would not return until I heard her call out nicely and asked for me to help her, no matter how long she stayed in there and screamed. I wrote my name on a piece of paper for her. I let her know it was her call. Then I walked out, shut the door, and waited. I didn't permit anyone else to go in the room. It took about a half an hour of what sounded like self-administered torture in the room before she asked for help, which she then got. She permitted an exam, she got IV fluids, she got an epidural, she quieted down, and she got a healthy baby. It was just not easy.

One night at 5PM I came on call to the Labor and Delivery deck as Chief obstetrical resident for the evening to find a busy labor floor with 8 patients in labor, and a woman in the corner room of the labor and delivery suite, apparently in that labor room all day and cared for by other residents during the day. She was in her early third trimester and in and out of lucidity all day. She had a psychiatric history, and the staff had been waiting all day for a psychiatric consultation to come and evaluate her. Almost exactly at 5 PM when the shift changed and I was now in charge, she went into shock with monitors beeping and blaring. There were no signs of outward bleeding, but the fetus was now in serious distress as well. A quick exam revealed her abdomen to be distended with no bowel sounds, vital signs unstable, in apparent hemorrhagic shock. I quickly placed her legs up and out, and placed a needle and syringe into her abdominal cavity through the vagina. It returned fresh blood from the abdominal cavity. The young woman was now in cardiac arrest. A stat code was called, IV's were started, blood and heart medication were administered, she was intubated and rushed to the operating room where an emergency surgery was performed to attempt arrest of the heavy internal bleeding from a ruptured cornual pregnancy, a form of ectopic pregnancy growing outside of the uterine cavity at the juncture of the tube and uterus. These abnormal pregnancies, rare and catastrophic, often will grow unnoticed until late in gestation before rupturing with resultant hemorrhage. It was the first and only time I ever did surgery on a patient in cardiac arrest, but it was a last and belated attempt to save her. If bleeding and vital signs could be stabilized, there was a slim chance of saving her life. It took me about five minutes to do an emergency hysterectomy, the fastest surgery I have ever done in my life. What the residents caring for her had assumed was a 'psych' patient because of her varying states of consciousness and ramblings during the day turned out to be a woman going in and out of consciousness due to blood loss and shock. She subsequently died on the operating table. This was just about the worst situation one could walk into to begin a night on call, but one never knows when the need to perform an emergency Cesarean Section or Cesarean hysterectomy will be necessary. Disasters like this were fortunately few and far between for both patient and physician, but always lurked around the corner in the world of obstetrics, which in a teaching hospital served to remind us all to be ever vigilant, a lesson none of us every forgot.

Obesity is just a bad thing. No two ways about

it. No matter what causes it, no matter why a person is obese, it only serves to make their own lives shortened and worse than whatever else life would have been for them. And it certainly doesn't make it easier as a physician to deal with obese patients. But in medicine, as in cards, one has to learn to deal the hand one is dealt. One patient came into Labor and Delivery during residency weighing somewhere between 500-550 pounds, best guess, since there was no way to weigh her. She said she had prenatal care elsewhere, but certainly not in our clinic and we were unable to retrieve any records. If she hadn't told us she was pregnant and in labor we would not have known. We were able to pick up an occasional fetal heart tone with an external Doppler ultrasound device, but were unable to pick up anything with fetal monitoring. When it came time to examine her in the labor bed, I put on a sterile glove, pulled down the sheet and asked her to let her legs drop to the side. She told me they already were. Instantly I knew I was in trouble now since I couldn't even see the vagina to do a cervical exam. There were layers of thigh fat obscuring the view. So I began to dig my way in, moving the thigh fat to the side with the assistance of nurses on each side to further retract her inner thighs. Eventually I could see the external vagina, but could not get my arm or hand near enough to get into the vagina, let alone up to the cervix for a pelvic exam, and she could not drop her legs to the side any further. It was futile. Kudos to the baby's father, whoever that was! Since she was reasonably comfortable, her vital signs were stable, and we could not monitor her on the fetal monitor, we sent her away from the labor floor to a regular post partum bed to wait more regular contractions before we brought her back. About 30 minutes after she arrived to her regular bed we got a stat call to run up to her room. After one push I found a five-pound healthy baby between her legs and the rolls of fat. Some people are just lucky.

What a contrast of experiences one sees at a teaching hospital! One lady, again in the 500-pound range and a patient of our obstetrical clinic during residency, was scheduled for a repeat Cesarean section. She was brought to the operating room and prepared for surgery. The anesthesiologist had opted to administer a regional anesthetic, or spinal, rather than a general anesthetic with intubation that he had determined to be riskier in her case. After a difficult and valiant attempt at the spinal, he laid her on her back in preparation for surgery, and while she was having her abdomen prepped she began to have a grand mal seizure, likely a result of the spinal medication. I had a 500-pound woman in front of me seizing on the operating table with a baby inside of her that we could not monitor. The table and literally the room were shaking in rhythm with her as she seized. All we could do was try to keep her on the table without injuring herself. Mindful of the first rule of medicine, "Primum non nocere" or "Do no harm", I could not do a stat Cesarean section on her until she herself had been stabilized, which everyone around her was working so hard to do. When the patient was finally in stable condition, intubated and medicated to stop the seizures, only then could I begin the surgery. Cutting through that many layers of adipose tissue (fat) is always an experience. Much like a knife going through butter, it begins rather easily, but then as one incises further and further deep into the adipose tissue, one realizes how much further down are the other layers of the abdomen, the muscle, the fascia, the peritoneum, the uterus, and then the baby. It was like digging a ditch with a scalpel. In this situation it is not something one can rush through. I had no idea what shape the baby was going to be in, but I was not about to jeopardize the mother's life. As luck would have it, the baby was in good condition, and all turned out well for the Mom. But what a huge layer of risk she added to her life, and that of her child.

Lucky, too, was a patient of mine who walked into my office one day in Phoenix, a first time Mom near her due date. I can still picture her walking down the hall way with that uncomfortable open leg waddle most term pregnant patients have, one hand behind her back. I greeted her, asked how she was doing, and she replied great, but that she wasn't sure what was going on and just wanted to come in for a checkup. My nurse put her in the exam room, got her into a gown, and told her I would be right in. I came in about five minutes later and chatted with her, and then said, "OK, time for an exam". She put her legs comfortably in the stirrups. I proceeded to examine her, and ran smack into the baby's head sitting right on the perineum ready for delivery. We had an emergency delivery kit in the office that my nurse hurriedly retrieved. I had her push once, and out slid a healthy baby girl. Everyone in the office was excited, especially the other women in the waiting room as we wheeled her through with the newborn in her lap on the way to the hospital. I am sure most of the women waiting said, "If she could do that, so can I". I just never saw it happen before or after, but she totally missed her labor. Good for her. Lucky.

As a new obstetrician on staff at my hospital in Phoenix I was clearly being observed carefully by the nursing staff who of course wanted to know what the new kid on the block had to offer, and whether they were comfortable with me. First impressions were important. Before the first week passed, I was indeed dismayed to find that the first three pregnant patients that I managed did not make it to the delivery room. One in fact delivered hurriedly in the emergency department before she ever got to the Labor and Delivery suite. One was an emergency Cesarean section and delivered in the operating room, and the third was a late spontaneous miscarriage also handled in the emergency department. I felt as if the staff were wondering if I would ever get someone to the Labor and Delivery suite. But that quickly passed as I settled in and the nursing staff came to know me better. I always did as much teaching as I could, and always had the family practice residents at my side since I frequently supervised them on their own patients and let them deliver many of my own. In those early days at the 250-bed community hospital in Arizona adjacent to our office, I felt like I had taken a step backwards from the high tech teaching institution from where I had come in Pennsylvania. The equipment was outdated as were the monitors, the facility was old and in serious need of updating and modernization, there was no NICU, and epidurals were not being given. In fact, I was the only obstetrician on staff trained to give epidurals. If a patient wanted one, the anesthesiologist would have to be called in, often in the middle of the night, and they were reluctant to come and sit with the patient for hours until they delivered. So I just took to administering my own epidurals again, which everyone advised me against in the fear that something would go wrong since I had no back up. But I did so for the first few years. I was trained to do so and comfortable doing so. I eventually became chairman of the OB-GYN department, and set up an epidural program whereby epidurals were administered by nurse anesthetists and supervised by anesthesiologists.

The old adage applied that if you want something done right do it yourself.

One weekend when I was on call, a new patient whom I had only seen once in the office, with her husband in tow, came into Labor and Delivery in active labor on Sunday afternoon. I was at home and got a call from the OB nurse about her arrival, but with the comment that her husband said if I was on call and came in to the hospital and touched his wife he was going to kill me. I had no idea what his problem was, but she needed attention, and I was it for the day. He demanded another Doctor be called to care for his laboring wife. I made an attempt to find someone else who would care for these people. Not surprisingly I was unsuccessful. Asking someone to give up a Sunday afternoon to care for a patient with a violent husband was met with expected resistance from others. I informed the nurse I was on my way in but that she was to get hospital security and have him removed from the labor suite first. When I arrived I saw this gentleman from the rear, wearing a cowboy hat and snake skinned boots glancing over his shoulders at me while being forcibly hauled off by two armed security guards. He muttered rather loudly that he would kill me some day. He was distraught about something. She turned out to be very nice and had an uneventful delivery. Forcibly removing someone from the labor room was not my thing but I saw no other way to deal with it in this case.

The next day in the Doctor's lunch room at the hospital, with this episode fresh in mind, I went through the food line and sat at a table with a good dozen or so physicians who were eating their lunch, heavy into a conversation about guns. I listened for a while as I ate my spaghetti and meatballs. They were into a heavy discussion about guns and gun laws in Arizona, and it became clear to me that most of these physicians owned guns. I chimed into the conversation at the right time and asked how many of them owned guns. Every single one of them, surgeons, cardiologists, pathologists, anesthesiologists, obstetricians, pediatricians all owned a handgun. For someone that never owned a gun and never permitted my kids to have anything other than one squirt gun for backyard pool play, I was astounded. I then asked if they would all use the gun to shoot someone if necessary, and again it was unanimous. These were physicians, sworn to care for the sick and injured, Good Samaritans. If every one of them had and would use a handgun then everyone in Arizona had at least one gun-except me, that is. I was stunned and obviously the odd man out. But this was America, it was the Wild West in Arizona, and it was a fact of life, like it or not.

Another time when I found myself raising my voice was with a longstanding patient of mine. She was an intelligent and mature woman, however consumed with many neuroses. Her care was not easy and often required extensive reassurance that there was nothing wrong with her and she would be alive and well next year when she came in for her annual exam. Then she got pregnant with twins, and I cared for her for nine months, which went remarkably well despite all the neuroses. She chose not to see any of my partners. She had a birth plan that we went over ad nauseam to satisfy her needs. Of course when she went into labor the birth plan went out the window, and all her inner fears came unhinged the whole time she was in labor. When she finally got into the delivery room, she was unglued, unable to control herself or her movements, arms and legs flailing, swearing at the top of her lungs and jeopardizing the healthy birth of her twins since she could not be examined. Her husband was with her and utterly dismayed and embarrassed, but stunningly silent. I expect he had never seen her like this. Delivery of twins can be complicated depending on their position and time between birth. It was not a time for her to be out of control, especially after 9 months of us reviewing things on multiple occasions. So again, with the labor and delivery nurses and her husband in the room, I shut the door and had a 'face to face' conversation with her. The nurses backed against the wall. Underneath their surgical masks which covered their nose and mouth I could see their eyes widen with both surprise, because they had never seen me talk like this to anyone before, and joy, because they thought she deserved everything I was saying. I told her she was acting like an immature baby, worse than what I would expect of her and that I would not accept any responsibility for her safety or the safety of her unborn twins unless she listened to me and cooperated. I asked her husband to sign a medical release form. And I would walk out until she asked nicely for me to return. I was amazed at how effective this technique was the few times I was forced to use it, and quickly adopted if for my own kids when all else failed. Even the nurses were impressed. When someone never hears you talk with a raised voice, it is stunning when it happens and often brings people to listen intently to what is being said. Do it all the time and it will not command respect. The few times when my kids saw me angry, they listened, too. For this patient, in the end all went well and she was most apologetic when she returned to the office several weeks later, with two healthy twins in tow.

Instrumental vaginal deliveries require special skill, expertise, and knowledge of the limits of a normal labor and delivery, when intervention is necessary, and when one's own strength can be injurious to the baby. Choosing the kind of intervention required, the length of time one safely attempts the instrumental delivery, and when to bail after having failed in favor of a Cesarean Section is critical to the good outcome of birth for both mother and child. By instrumental vaginal deliveries I mean that a patient has gotten to the point of complete dilatation of the cervix, she has pushed effectively and for sufficient time so that her powers of pushing and the powers of labor are no longer effective. Intervention becomes necessary because the baby will no longer come out on its own or with the mother's help. Thus delivery needs to be effected by an obstetrician.

One's judgment, experience and expertise now come into play. The options are vacuum assisted vaginal delivery, forceps delivery, or operative delivery by Cesarean section. Each requires knowledge of a number of things; maternal bony pelvis size and shape, size of the baby, exact position of the baby's head, an empty bladder, and a seated obstetrician from which not too much force can be applied.

As with most vignettes I have recounted, it is only the outlying cases that one tends to remember and which stand out. My first week as an intern started two weeks before the Chief Residents at the time finished their four-year program. One day one of the Chief's was performing a difficult forceps rotation, a forceps delivery that not only required traction but rotation of the fetal head with the forceps in place, a difficult and potentially dangerous maneuver for both mother and baby. He was an enormous, overweight guy, and word quickly spread on the Labor and Delivery floor that he was having trouble. Many of the new residents gathered outside the labor room behind closed doors and peered through a window into the delivery room, which afforded us a view of his seated body in front of the mother. His scrubs were tight and short, and in the seated position we could all see more of his butt than was attractive. More interesting was the force he was using to pull on the forceps, an impressive site on its own. And yet there was no movement of the baby's head despite his forceful efforts. He pulled mightily on numerous occasions. I was frightened just watching but assumed at the time this was normal since ostensibly he knew what he was doing and I didn't. At just one of these moments, for reasons still hard to fathom, the forceps handles, which lock in place when applied to the baby's head, came disengaged while he was pulling. He rolled backwards off the stool and fell against the wall, the heavy metal forceps hit the floor with a clang, and I looked around the room to find the baby's head, assuming incorrectly that he had pulled it off. There was a stunned hush that went up amongst those of us watching. What a site to have seen though, never before, never since, but I developed a healthy lifelong respect for forceps deliveries from that day forward.

There are two scenarios in Obstetrics that one has lifelong nightmares about with the hope that one never finds one's self in such a situation. If there, though, one needs to know what to do since they are both obstetrical emergencies that may result in death of the baby or permanent injury. The first scenario is called a shoulder dystocia. The shoulders of a delivering baby can get stuck in the maternal bony pelvis such that the head has delivered and is outside of the vagina, but the shoulders remain hung up in the bony pelvis and the rest of the body doesn't deliver. Once this occurs, the obstetrician has an obstetrical emergency on his or her hands with time being of the essence. There are obstetrical maneuvers that one must know how to perform rather quickly to deliver the baby. Time quickly becomes a factor in this scenario since although the head is out, the chest is not, so breathing is not yet possible due to chest compression, and oxygen no longer gets to the baby because the umbilical cord is trapped in the vagina and compressed, cutting off oxygen. Fetal hemoglobin is forgiving in a sense because it will hold onto oxygen for a good five minutes before brain damage occurs. Five minutes seems like a long time or a short time depending on one's frame of reference, but to an obstetrician sitting on the delivery stool, in this scenario, it goes by pretty quickly, especially if all the maneuvers one is trained to do are not working. One tends to panic, pull too hard and quickly in an effort to get the baby out, and can result in delivery but with a damaged arm from stretching of the nerves in the neck. So one must avoid traction in this scenario, a very hard thing to resist even though it is one's gut instinct to do so with time ticking away. Maneuvers must be repeated in sequence, and often repeated again, all designed to effect delivery without excessive traction. One night while my wife and I were having dinner with two of our resident friends in their apartment nearby the hospital, one of the chief residents got a stat call to run to the hospital for just such an emergency that was happening on the labor floor. When he returned about an hour later, he related the sad outcome. The baby's head had been delivered and despite everyone's best efforts and maneuvers, the baby suffocated because none of the maneuvers were successful at freeing up the impacted shoulders. He was as white as a ghost when he returned and I don't think he ever completely recovered from this nightmare. And of course even though I was not there, I could only imagine this happening to me someday. One tends to scrupulously avoid ever getting in this situation and to always remember the risk factors that predispose to being in this situation – an excessively large baby or mother, a dysfunctional labor that is not progressing properly, a difficult instrumental delivery which is not going well, a diabetic mom with a large baby and large estimated fetal weight, among others. One never forgets the maneuvers that must be applied in rapid succession to free the baby's shoulders up and effect delivery. This scenario has been the cause of many malpractice suits due to permanent damage that frequently will occur to the baby's shoulder and arm, causing it to wither over time from muscular atrophy secondary to the damaged nerves. Many courtroom arguments exist over what is too much traction, how it was applied, what maneuvers were attempted, what caused this horrible outcome and whether it could have been avoided.

The second nightmare scenario is a breech delivery with a trapped fetal head.

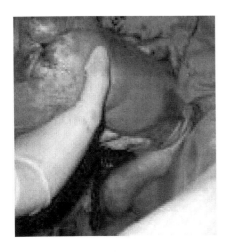

In a breech delivery the baby's bottom comes out first, then the body, with the head last. The baby's head is the largest part of the body, and it is bony as opposed to the soft body. When a baby comes head first, if the head comes out, the body follows with ease. When faced with a breech delivery, the body will always come out since it is smaller and softer than the head, but if the head gets stuck in the maternal bony pelvis, one is faced with a body in hand, and a head still in the maternal bony pelvis, an untenable and often life ending situation for the fetus. So nightmares abound surrounding breech deliveries. I was trained in the day that still allowed us as obstetricians to do breech deliveries. The reality is that the large majority of them go smoothly if selected properly, the labor monitored closely, and the maneuvers to deliver a breech baby are carefully followed. But selection and experience are critical. Make a mistake here and a nightmare scenario follows. That is why today most obstetricians will simply just do a Cesarean section if the baby is breech either because they have never been trained to do a breech vaginal delivery, or are just too scared to even attempt one. But I was from the old school where we did attempt them and successfully complete them when selected properly, although there was always risk involved until the head was out. Imagine then the horror of watching one of my attending physicians during residency faced with a breech delivery, the feet out, and looking at a foot that was probably half the size of mine (perhaps an exaggeration, but that is how large it was, and over the years seems to have even gotten larger in my dreams). An audible gasp went up in the delivery room when everyone saw the size of the foot that portended a huge baby and even larger head. He obviously had not selected this patient well, for had he estimated the fetal weight correctly or had assessed the other risk factors properly, would not have found himself in this position. Fortunately for him, he performed the breech maneuvers quickly and effectively, and even more fortunately for him the mother had a huge bony pelvis with ample room. A 13-pound baby came out, the largest I have ever seen, without damage. But the nightmare persists to this day. I have performed many vaginal breech deliveries because selection was a key lesson I learned, and knowing what a normal labor versus an abnormal one looks like, as well as becoming good at estimating fetal weight and evaluating risk factors. Many of today's obstetricians have never seen or performed a breech delivery and just opt for a Cesarean section, which of course increases the Cesarean section rate and maternal risk. But everyone has a different level of skill and comfort with situations that Mother Nature presents, and if one is uncomfortable with handling a situation either because of lack of training or fear, a Cesarean section is a better option in order to avoid a catastrophe. No argument from me on that one. Skills change. Experience varies. Teaching programs differ. The ability to handle stressful situations varies from human being to human being. Thus the art of obstetrics changes over the years.   What doesn't change is the constant state of exhaustion.

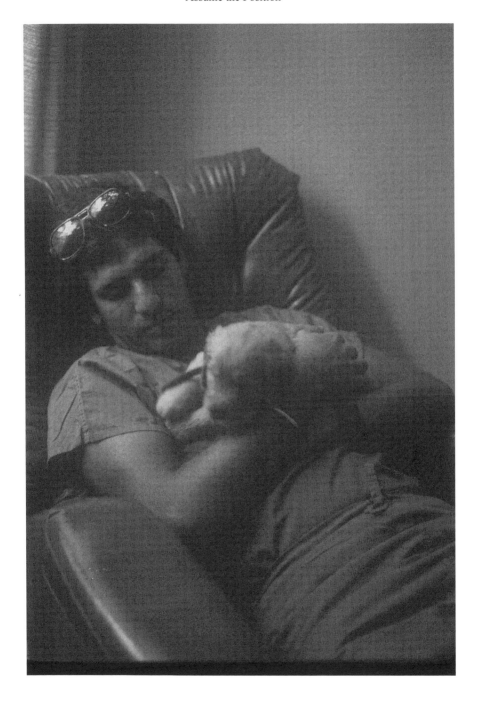

Chapter 4   Office Life

Behind every office door was a new and different patient, and a new emotional situation; an obstetrical patient in for her first visit with her significant other (joy, delight, excitement and apprehension); a newly pregnant patient unhappy about being so and requesting an abortion (sadness, determination, confusion, embarrassment, apathy); an infertility patient unable to conceive (worry, fear, depression, hope, disappointment); a third trimester pregnant patient (discomfort, anxiety, impatience); a newly diagnosed case of genital

herpes (anger, pain, disbelief); a woman
requesting permanent sterilization(relief and
gratitude);abnormal uterine bleeding (frustration
and fear);a breast lump (fear); pelvic pain (pain);
contraception(relief and freedom); hot flashes
(hormonal changes).   And so the day went, day
after day. Not only were skills called into play to
make the proper diagnosis, make
recommendations, prescribe medications, offer
surgery when necessary and appropriate, allow
freedom of choice for continued hormonal and
reproductive health, but also counseling skills
were required with almost every single patient,
even if nothing other than reassurance that the
situation and complaint were well within the
norms. Of course, emotions within me would rise
and fall all day long, but keeping emotions in
check and compartmentalized was an important,
and difficult part of maintaining objectivity so
that I could offer my patients the best advice
available under the circumstances. For me this is
what made the day interesting, challenging,
difficult and exciting. The patient schedule
produced for me each day simply had a name

and time. It gave no clue as to what I was going to walk into when I opened the exam room door.

Many people would often question how a man could understand and be sensitive to the complaints, trials and tribulations of an Obstetrical and Gynecologic patient. Clearly one does not need to be a woman to be able to empathize and be sensitive. After all, as a physician, does one need to have cancer to be able to be sensitive to a cancer patient? I have found over the years that women physicians are no more able to empathize with a female patient than a male physician. In fact, many of our friends and patients would complain to me about the attitudes of some of the female practitioners in my office or others. Rather than the gender of the physician, what is more important is the empathic and sensitive nature of the physician, something that is not inherent only to the X chromosome, even if one has two XX chromosomes.

I had an unusual ability to pick up the chart from outside the door, see the name on it, and pretty much be able to recall the patient's history regardless of time interval between visits, and visualize the patient's face before I opened the door. If I passed the patient in the mall the next week, or saw her in Price Club, I could not recall her name or the details of the exam or problem which was often vexing for me because patients of course remembered me and expected me to remember them, their deliveries, their surgeries, their children, etc. But because I devoted intense individual attention to each patient when they were in front of me, then dictated my office note as soon as I walked out of the exam room, everything seemed to erase itself from my mind when I shut off the Dictaphone and turned attention to the next patient, until I saw the chart on the door the next time they were in the office. This practice required detailed dictation with notes to myself for the next time the patient would appear in the office. When I was in the exam room with the patient everyone received my undivided attention, and I never left the room without first asking if there were any other questions that needed to be answered. I found that most patients were hesitant and afraid to ask questions, so I needed to tap into their fears, anticipate them, and deal with them before they left the office, which I accepted as my mission for every single office visit, no matter how long it might take. If someone needed more time, they got it. If it was an easy routine matter or annual exam, I offered reassurance and quickly moved on so as not to keep the next patient waiting. Every examination required differing amounts of time. I hated to keep scheduled patients waiting, although of necessity it happened depending on the amount of time each problem would take. I would also sit myself down on the stool and stay there until all questions were asked and answered. If a detailed conversation were necessary, such as a surgery had to be discussed in detail and options given, I would ask the patient to get dressed and come into my consultation room with whomever they brought with them for a further detailed discussion. I preferred to keep patients waiting in the waiting room than in the exam room. Thus there were never more than two patients at a time in my exam rooms; the one I was seeing, and the next patient getting ready with my nurse giving her instructions on my behalf, checking urine, vital signs, logging in the complaint, readying the exam room, laying out the gown and Pap smear, etc. Thus I could quickly move from one room to the other, and then back again after completing the dictation. I was constantly looking at my watch outside of the exam room because I hated to keep patients waiting, and tried my best to stick to the schedule. Time was important to the patient as well. The business being what it was, however, often caused delays in the schedule, whether because of frequent trips to the labor and delivery suite (there was almost always someone in labor who also required attention at unpredictable times), a phone call that couldn't wait for some reason or another, etc. Many days there just weren't enough hours in the day to get everything accomplished, which in itself created pressures.

Hospital rounds were made first thing in the morning, before the OR schedule and before office hours, so usually at 6 or 6:30 AM. It was a good time to make rounds on patients because all was usually quiet in the hospital then, there were usually few interruptions before the day got busy, and I could get through rounds efficiently, or if needed, had time to deal with any post operative complications should they arise. One never quite knew what was going to be found on morning rounds. Post operative fevers, wound infections, bleeding, unexpected complications, inadequate pain control were some of the more common but infrequent problems. On weekends I would make rounds on my partner's patients when I was on call and while they were off. I always volunteered to work on Christmas day because it wasn't my holiday so that partners could spend time with their families. I remember very well one Christmas day early on hospital rounds when I walked in to see a woman who was on her first post operative day, my partner having done a major abdominal surgery on her the day before. I cheerily said " Good morning". She replied, " Are you Jewish?" " Yes ", I said. She continued on: " You are going to burn in hell". I took a moment to think what to say next, but not too long, then replied:" You should worry about where you are going, and I will worry about where I am going". I had trouble seeing the Christian spirit in her greeting that morning. I am a bit ashamed to say that when I removed her bandage, I should have done it a bit more slowly than I did. But religious discrimination just didn't sit pretty with me that morning.

All my surgeries usually started at 7:30 in the morning, sharp. This required making hospital rounds on delivered or post operative patients before surgery started, often requiring me to leave home by 6 AM daily, or if sleeping in the hospital because of a laboring patient, to arise and start rounds then. No matter what, I had to find time for a morning shower before starting the day to put me in synchrony with my biorhythms. Among other things, it cleared the air and seemed like it gave me a fresh start to the day, even if I had been up all night. The operating room nurses knew that I was pretty demanding about a 7:30 major abdominal or vaginal operation starting at 7:30. AM. After all, it was the first case of the day and there really was no excuse for it starting at 8:00 because people were dragging their feet – or so I saw it. Most of my cases could be completed by 9:00 so that I could start office hours promptly unless I had a delivery. My main office was adjacent to the hospital where I did most of my deliveries so as not to waste time riding around the city in my car or rushing to get somewhere and risking an accident. Frequently I would do minor surgeries over the noon hour since they were less time consuming. Then back to the office for an afternoon of patients and business. It was a full and exhausting day often followed by night call! Efficiency and time management were critical and routine for me.

We had a very interesting waiting room. We cared for patients from all walks of life; the upper crust from Scottsdale and Paradise Valley; the uninsured poverty stricken from inner city Phoenix; White, Hispanic, Native American, young and old; hopefuls who couldn't conceive, and those who could but didn't want to; those who had previously had abortions, and those who had no idea we did pregnancy terminations. Everyone sat next to each other, and everyone was treated exactly alike. Everyone also had one thing in common -two X chromosomes. There was nothing we could or should do about controlling conversation in the waiting room. I found the waiting room a wonderful, egalitarian place where women came for good medical care. Not everyone cared for the patient mixture. I suppose those who didn't like sitting next to someone for some reason just didn't come back. So be it. Those who wanted to be there kept coming; those that didn't went elsewhere.

My practice was a group practice. When I joined it I was the third physician in the group and we all worked out of one small office. Over the years the practice grew tremendously, became a group of 10 physicians including four nurse midwives and physician assistants, with the addition of three other offices around the city, and staff privileges at five different hospitals. There was only one business office for the whole group that was located across the hall from the main office where I worked. Each of the other offices was located adjacent to one of the other hospitals so that no one had to be driving around during the day.

It was important for the patients to be able to choose which physician in the group practice they wanted to see as their primary physician. Gynecologic patients would stay with their primary physician unless the physician was out of town or there was an emergency, and then would be seen by whoever else was available. Obstetrical patients were requested to see the other physicians at least once so that they would be familiar with each doctor should that doctor be on call when they came in during labor. Patients then could choose to return to see their favorite physician at the office of their choosing at their next appointment.

Concessions had to be made to accommodate physician life style and good medical practice. The physicians all had a day off. We all had vacation time, so we all needed to cover for each other at various times, and we all needed to practice medicine in a similar fashion. Therefore, dictated typed notes with treatment plans were essential for a number of reasons, not the least of which was readability but also so we could follow each other's prescribed treatment plans.

As the practice grew and expanded with a rapidly growing city, we continued to add new physicians. My original two partners and I were East Coast males trans-located to Phoenix. When it came time to add a fourth physician, we purposely sought out a female physician for diversity, thinking she would become busy immediately from our overflow and her gender. We were mistaken. Most of the women in our practice only wanted to see a male physician and were not comfortable seeing a woman, a surprise to us. After all that is why they were already coming to the practice. So it took some time for the new female physician to get as busy as the rest of us, which in due course did happen as she developed her own clientele from new patients we put in front of her. When we next expanded, the best recruit was an African American man, so we offered him a position. We thought this might be a difficult transition for our patients, but again we were wrong. He was busy from day one, mostly because of his winning personality and demeanor. The only patient I ever asked to leave our practice was a long time patient of the practice, newly pregnant, who refused to see our newest associate because of his skin color. I sat the patient down one day to discuss the situation, and explain that there was a possibility he could deliver her since we rotated night call for our own mental and physical health. She refused to even sit in the same room with him. I explored her fears with her. Apparently her family was from inner city Detroit, had a small mom and pop grocery store, and her parents were robbed and brutalized by a gang on more than one occasion. She not only was prejudiced against all African Americans, but also would not even sit in the same room with him. I explained to her that he was extremely competent, nice, gentle and caring. She adamantly refused even to sit across the desk with him for a discussion. I told her to think long and hard about it, and call me back, but that if she couldn't' speak to him human being to human being, she would have to receive care elsewhere. She never returned.

Our office décor was quite upscale, nicely furnished, carpeted, with comfortable seating in the waiting room. There was extensive artwork and warm inviting colors throughout. We had a beautiful saltwater fish tank that was the first thing visible to people as they went from the waiting room back to the exam rooms. The fish were our 'babies' and required a lot of daily care and love. But they were beautiful. After all, it was a good sign if we could keep fish alive, not always as easy as it might otherwise appear in a saltwater tank.

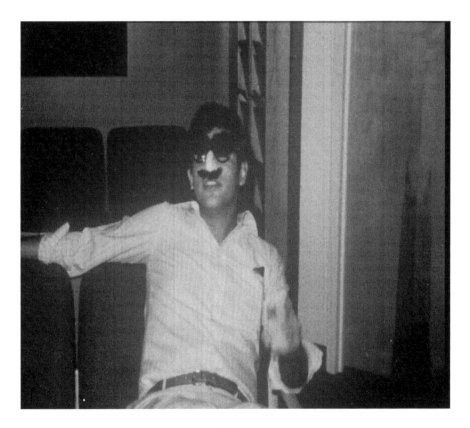

(Halloween in the office was always a fun time.)

   Life in Arizona was good to us. I was busy and the medical practice flourished. As if we didn't' have enough to do, one of my partners and I established Women's Health Research of Arizona which kept us on the forefront of new developments in the specialty. We tested multiple FDA sponsored protocols for clinical trials testing new medications and procedures in Obstetrics and Gynecology. I had several articles published in medical journals all referable to a new in-office sterilization procedure we had begun to perform. The clinical research kept us in the forefront of emerging medicine in the field, and we developed a local and national reputation for innovation. My partner and I frequently travelled to give lectures, attend investigator meetings, and make presentations to other OB GYN physicians. Scrupulous record keeping was essential since the FDA could appear at any time, and frequently did, to audit our charts to make sure everything we were doing was in compliance with their protocols. It also necessitated having a full time nurse coordinator for both patient education and care in these investigative studies. It was challenging, interesting work, new medicine that was not yet taught in medical schools or residency programs. In fact, we had resident physicians from throughout Arizona often spend time with us for weeks at a time to see procedures and techniques for treatment of abnormal bleeding that in their hands and those of other private practitioners would result in a hysterectomy. Teaching was just a routine part of the day, every day. However, in our hands these patients could be handled either in office or in a short outpatient surgical procedure with the patient going back to work the next day without major surgery, a major clinical advancement for the patients.

I found that brutal honesty was often the best way to deal with unpleasant diagnoses. Most patient's could understand and appreciate bad news if delivered forthrightly without sugar coating, deal with the emotion in whatever time needed to clear the air, and then the discussion could begin with all the options presented in a step wise fashion. It was a strange set of circumstances that caused me to deliver my first cancer diagnosis to my own father. While early in my second year of medical school, my dad developed a problem that was not being managed well by his local physician. I implored him to come to Philadelphia to see my professor of Urology at Hahnemann, which resulted in a biopsy on a Thursday afternoon. Saturday morning he and I were waiting all morning in his hospital room for the Professor to make rounds and deliver the biopsy diagnosis, but for some reason he was delayed. I went out of the room to the nurse's station to inquire his whereabouts and found the Professor's resident also sitting

and waiting for the urologist to come. He
informed me of the diagnosis – prostate cancer. I
guess I was gone for five minutes or so and then
came back into my dad's room. He asked me
what I found out. I could have simply lied and
said 'nothing,' the doctor will be here soon,
which would have been the easy way out. But
despite my discomfort, I chose to tell him the
truth. He handled it quite well, perhaps because
he expected as much, perhaps because he could
read my face. Once one tells their parents an
unpleasant diagnosis, nothing else is particularly
difficult after that. So for me, I learned the lesson
and the technique early on. Straightforward
honesty and truth delivered with sensitivity gets
the job done.

Nothing, however, was as difficult for me as
having to tell a pregnant patient who presented
to the office complaining of lack of fetal
movement that she had a dead baby inside of
her. In most cases where expectant Mom's feel
lack of movement, it is usually short lived and a

quick ultrasound in the office confirms a good heartbeat and all is well. But there were those times when the patient would be lying on the ultrasound table, watching the fetal monitor with me awaiting my reassurance. Although I could tell instantly the baby was not living because I knew where to look for the heart beat, the mother would not know as fast as I would. It was always a difficult few seconds having this knowledge before the apprehensive patient who was anxiously lying in front of me. I would use the time to scan some more and to collect my thoughts and anticipate how best to deliver the news to the particular patient, all of whom took the news the same way – disbelief, shock, tears, sadness. Many patients would question whether or not I was sure, and of course I would never deliver that news if I weren't. It just didn't get easier over time, and was one of the worst parts of the specialty. These obstetrical accidents happened, fortunately rarely, and there was never fault attached although most patients would begin by trying to blame themselves. Hugs, hand holding and a quiet period of reflection were usually helpful; I would wait for the patient to speak first, then begin the process of answering her questions and discussing what the next steps were.

Infertility patients presented their own set of emotional and gynecologic problems all of which needed to be dealt with in an orderly fashion. The first issue at hand was of course a complete history and physical exam to help ascertain whether the medical definition of infertility was indeed met, or whether the patient just needed to go back out and keep trying, or whether correcting anything with a simple discussion was all that was necessary. Blame to one partner or the other had already been assigned in most cases before the patient ever arrived at the office, however incorrectly. Some people just assumed that having intercourse six times a day was all that was necessary, which was of course part of the problem. Others simply needed to stop using contraception. Others needed to understand the menstrual cycle and when fertility was highest. Others needed to return with the husband in tow and the investigation would begin there. Everyone needed to produce a sperm specimen for analysis before anything else was done. The reality is that the male system is relatively easy to investigate. If a man were producing sperm with an adequate sperm count, and putting it in the right place, which interestingly wasn't always the case, often his investigation would end; conversely, if the sperm count was inadequate, he needed a more detailed urological evaluation. The female reproductive system is much more complex, and needs a stepwise evaluation including a menstrual history, ovulatory history, an examination for anatomical abnormalities, hormonal and blood tests, tubal patency and x-rays, and occasionally a laparoscopic or hysteroscopic exam of the internal female anatomy. It was often a laborious and time consuming evaluation, but when the cause was ascertained, male or female or occasionally both, it often could be corrected to the utter joy of the patient, some of the happiest and most loyal patients one could ever hope for.

Of course, all kinds of fears had to be
addressed in the office setting, perhaps none of
which caused more apprehension for most
people than getting naked to some extent before
a complete stranger. This of course applies to
physicians as well, since we, too, become
patients from time to time, and find ourselves
similarly exposed. But a woman getting naked in
front of a strange man is a unique set of
circumstances that requires sensitivity and
understanding. We always had long cloth gowns
that served much as a bathrobe, and gave the
patient some sense of dignity. I would always
meet a fully clothed new patient in my office first
for her medical history, then escort her into the
exam room and let my nurse explain the
disrobing and robing procedure. I would usually
give the patient several minutes before entering
the room, then upon entering the room begin
with a general physical exam, thyroid exam, listen
to the heart and lungs before doing a breast

exam and reserving the pelvic exam for last. When finished, I would begin a discussion with the patient seated on the table, and me seated on the exam stool, so that she was above me rather than me standing above her or leaning on the door like it was time for me to run out of the room and see someone else. I never gave the patient a sense that I had other things on my mind or needed to be somewhere else. Simply put, it was just common sense to do these things to put the patient at ease as much as possible.

For some people, however, no matter what one did to try to ease the discomfort of the situation, nothing was enough. Discomfort was also a two way street. When in medical school as a second year medical student, I was sent to Reading, Pennsylvania for my very first obstetrical and gynecologic rotation. As a second year medical student, I knew nothing about clinical medicine yet, having spent the entire first year in academic training and labs. We had practiced pelvic exam on latex pelvic models, but never on a live breathing human being with normal female pelvic anatomy staring me in the face. So I was petrified of my first pelvic exam. The attending physician with whom I was working was very liberal and sent me in for the history and exam unaccompanied. I found an attractive young woman sitting on the exam stool, leaning forward, robe open in the front with most of her breasts indiscreetly showing. She didn't seem to care one bit. I did my best not to be flustered and proceeded to find out that she was there for a routine exam. Lucky me, I could get this over with and get out of the room quickly. When she got her legs in the stirrups and she slid down to the end of the table, I proceeded to do the speculum exam as skillfully as I could without hurting her and as if I knew what I was doing. I then proceeded to perform a bimanual exam, with one gloved hand in the vagina and the other on the lower abdomen so as to be able to feel the pelvic organs (I really was just going through the motions and trying to get out of the room). I saw her hand slowly slide down over her abdomen and gently squeeze and massage my hand that was on her belly. I didn't know what to do or say, finished the exam and left the room. I never discussed what happened with the attending physician. He simply asked how it went and I said 'fine'. I had been petrified. She dressed, smiled at me on the way out, and left. It was amazing that this first pelvic exam, my first pelvic exam, began and ended this way. To this day, I have no idea whether he set me up, whether she set me up, whether they were in cahoots together, or whether she just wanted to hold my hand.

My office was on the fifth floor of a building across the parking lot from the hospital, so that when one looked through the small vertical windows of the exam room it was perfectly obvious that unless one was on five story stilts peering in the window from the outside parking lot, or was in their hospital bed across the way with binoculars, no one could see into the windows. Imagine my surprise one day when I walked into the exam room and found the room pitch black, lights out, and window blinds closed in broad daylight. I asked if Mrs. Jones was still in the room, and she said yes, then I asked if there was a problem. She replied she couldn't run the risk of anyone seeing her naked so she closed the blinds and turned off the lights. I asked her if she realized she was on the fifth floor and no one could see into the windows, and of course she said she was aware. She also didn't want me to see her naked. I had to gently explain to her that I couldn't examine her without being able to see, that she did have on a gown and drape across her lap which covered her, that I was a physician who was there to care for her, not look at her. She ultimately relented, the room lights came on, and we managed to get through it without too much further trauma.

Then there was the opposite extreme. One day in the midst of a busy office session a new young patient presented herself to me with complaints of a vaginal infection. I interviewed her fully clothed in my consultation room first as was my custom, then escorted her to an exam room where I asked her to disrobe, put on a gown and I would return in a few minutes. I performed an exam, and she did indeed have an infection for which I prescribed medication and off she went. Two days later she was back again with the same complaints of itching and discharge. Of course I always felt badly when someone returned for a recurring problem, and assumed my diagnosis was incorrect. A repeat exam, a new prescription and off she went again, only to return for a third time a few days later with the same complaints. Again, back in the exam room to await my return. She was asked to disrobe and put on a gown. Five minutes later I knocked on the exam room door and walked in to find her standing stark naked, bright lights on, robe folded on the exam table, smiling, facing me, with no attempt to cover up anything, not the usual course of events in my day. I now couldn't help but notice her youth, her appearance, her body, her demeanor, and I bolted. I asked my nurse to go in, tell her to get dressed, to leave, and never to come back. Of course I documented the whole episode thoroughly in the medical chart and forgot about it.

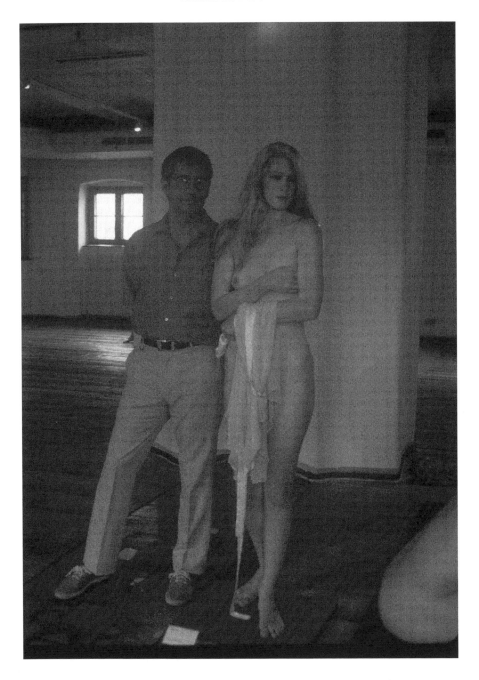

(I know you think this was the patient. Although
she looked similar, this photo was taken at a

museum in Vienna, Austria)

My nurse who had been with me for a number of years was top notch. Between the two of us we never missed anything. She knew my work habits well, the way I practiced and when and what I needed. We always had a professional relationship and I respected her contributions to my office life immensely. She often made my days easier just by anticipating my needs. About one month after the above episode, during a lunch hour when I was in my corner office with my feet on the desk reading a medical journal, there was a knock on my open inner office door. There was a young police woman standing there, a particularly shiny Phoenix police badge on her chest, gun in holster, and a piece of official looking paper in hand. She asked me to identify myself which I did then told me she had a summons for my arrest for sexual harassment of a patient. My heart sank to my ankles. I asked to see the summons that was very specific. Unable to even move my feet off the desk, I took time to read the summons, to think what I was going to do next and to catch my breath. I could feel the color drain from my face and my adrenaline pumping. I was regretting the fact that I rarely had a nurse with me in the exam room for routine exams unless a procedure of some sort was necessary. Psychogenic shock was beginning to set in. Whatever the charge was, I knew it wasn't true. My thoughts immediately went back to the young naked woman from a few weeks earlier. Just being charged by someone, however falsely, was enough to ruin my career. I told the officer there was a mistake. She told me she needed to handcuff me and take me to the station for formal charges. I told her there was no way I was being handcuffed and led out of my office. Her response was simple enough: "Are you resisting arrest?" I nodded affirmatively. Ultimately I chose not to resist as she handcuffed me and went to my desk. She picked up the desk phone and called her back up officer who immediately appeared. He had an electronic box of sorts which he placed on my desk and pressed a button. I was in semi panic mode, a place where I rarely if ever went. Music came on as she began to take off her clothes. My delighted office staff appeared from around the corner. They watched my horror in delight. Handcuffed at my desk I was about to receive a lap dance from the 'officer', now down to her skimpy panties and nothing else. I was in such shock that I couldn't even enjoy the experience, naked as she was and handcuffed as I was. Of course this occurred two days before my birthday, the furthest thing from my mind at that point. I never forgave my nurse for that one. I was a sitting duck and she got me. Such was life in an OB GYN office.

Shortly thereafter my front desk receptionist came to me and said, " There is a guy on the phone who wants to know if you would do a hysterectomy on him without seeing him in the office first." I looked at her like she was crazy. The answer was of course 'no' but I would be happy to see him if he thought he needed my services. So he made an appointment. When he arrived, balding and with a full beard, I learned he had been working as a male nurse for two years in a local hospital. He had been on male testosterone for that period of time and wanted 'his' uterus and ovaries removed. Thereafter he had plans with a plastic surgeon to have a bilateral simple mastectomy to remove his atrophied and hairy breasts that had been tightly bound. He then was moving to Seattle for a definitive surgery and a new life after a sex change operation. But first he wanted to get rid of his female organs. So I agreed and performed the abdominal surgery that usually required three days of hospitalization. After all it was a major surgical procedure. The first morning of surgical rounds I found him sitting bolt upright in a chair as if nothing had happened to him. He demanded to be discharged. I had never discharged anyone after this kind of surgery on the first post-operative day, because the intestines usually weren't ready for food yet, the pain was too intense from the abdominal incision, and people just weren't ready to move or even sit up. But I discharged him that day. As I subsequently tell the story for a laugh, I always used to say: "Well, he took it like a man!" The reality is that he took it like a very determined person. He was ready for the next phase of his life.

I had a patient who came in to me once with the complaint as follows: " My husband says I smell like a dead skunk that has been left in the desert for weeks on end". I wasn't sure what that smelled like, but I was accepting the statement as fact. She was put in the exam room and left waiting for me to enter. When I did, I was relieved that I honestly couldn't smell anything and then proceeded to examine her. When I placed the speculum in the vagina, I understood immediately what the problem was. High up in the vaginal vault were two tampons, one on top of the other. Evidently, two months earlier she had put in one last tampon at the end of her menstrual period, got drunk that night, and left the tampon in place for over a month, so that when she resumed her next period, she put in new tampons and never removed the old one through two menstrual cycles. Little choice but to remove it, put it in the trash can, thoroughly rinse the vagina with Betadine antiseptic and send her on her way. The real problem was after she left and my nurse came in the room to an overwhelming odor coming from the trashcan. The windows in the exam room didn't open. She wrapped up and closed the trash bag and took it way, and used most of a whole can of scented Lysol to try to get rid of the smell. The exam room was left unoccupied for the next several days until there was no trace whatsoever of the smell left, which is how long it took. So if one ever wonders what a dead skunk smells like that has been left in the desert for several days, you can now imagine!

And such was the office life of a busy Ob-GYN physician; never the same from one day to the next, or from one room to the next. Always interesting, unpredictable, challenging, and as varied as the women themselves.

Chapter 5 Night Life

Night call began during my second year of medical school. I couldn't wait to have my own beeper. It was a rite of passage and seemed to make me feel important that I was needed by someone in the middle of the night. I was eager to begin this phase of life about which there was often myth and mystery for the uninitiated medical student. The on call room for medical students at Hahnemann Medical College was on the 18th floor of the hospital, two floors above the inpatient psychiatric unit, and immediately above the hospital operators who were the ones calling us. It was always a thrill greeting the operators before retiring to the Spartan room with maybe a dozen beds, nothing more than a long dormitory room with a night stand and phone between every two beds. One could literally go all night without getting a call (rarely) and still have no sleep, since everyone else's phone was ringing even if mine wasn't. But ring they did. Medical students did 'scut work'; starting IV's, drawing blood and blood gases, putting Foley catheters into the bladder, and generally anything the interns and residents needed done that they wanted someone else to do for them so they could get some sleep. Hahnemann was unique in that rarely did anyone demonstrate how to do anything especially in the middle of the night. One was just supposed to figure it out or else ask the intern for help. But if one asked for help, our lack of knowledge would then be obvious and wound engender the response that if I wanted to do it myself, I would never have called you in the first place. Such was a big city teaching hospital. It was all part of the maturing experience.

No wonder then that when I was first called to put in my first Foley catheter into the bladder of an elderly female patient, I had no idea where the urethra was or how to insert the Foley. After an hour of torturing the poor woman, I finally implored the nurse to help me, which she willingly did. There was nothing like trying and failing, though, which served as a learning experience. It was humbling and traumatic to both the patient and to me. By the time we graduated medical school, however, we were clearly ready to be interns, without a doubt.

Internship and residency night call was a whole different ball of wax. The further one got in medical education, the fewer and fewer people there were to ask for advice, opinions and assistance, and the more one was expected to be able to handle problems on their own, especially at night time. The year I began my internship was July 1st, 1976, the bicentennial 200th anniversary of the United States. Pennsylvania Hospital, at 8th and Spruce streets in Philadelphia, was only a few blocks from all the celebration, Independence Hall, the Liberty Bell, and the Delaware River. It was the only hospital in the historical Society Hill section of Philadelphia. President Ford was in town, with thousands of others all crammed in to the same small area for the celebrations. The one assignment that I didn't want to begin my internship was my two-month stint in the Emergency Room as its intern; of course, that is what I got. Worse yet, my first shift was the late night shift that meant I was the only intern on that night in one of the busiest emergency rooms in the United States that evening. I was fully prepared, or so I thought, to handle whatever came in the door. I was the one who examined and triaged every single patient. There was clearly more advanced help available who would come if I called, but it was my call to determine if I could handle the situation or needed to call for help. In many respects, the hardest cases to manage were the ones that I sent home without anyone else seeing the patient but me. If someone was so sick that they needed hospitalization then I called for resident help. But making the determination that someone was not going to die or get worse if I sent them home with treatment was all on my shoulders. It was a great learning experience. I saw everything from asthma, to heart attacks, to gun shot wounds of the head, to maggot infested plaster leg casts, to nose bleeds, diabetic shock, toe nail hemorrhages, heart failure, and everything in between. I was forever grateful to the late night emergency room nurses, who knew much more than I did.

Residency night call was again a different experience. This was the beginning of obstetrics and gynecology learning. There were four residents in my year. This meant we were on call in the hospital every fourth night and every fourth weekend. There were four residents on call each night, one from each of the four years in the program, and we all had different workloads and decision-making responsibility. At one point, for several months, one of the women in my year developed vision problems, so we had to then cover every third night and third weekend.

"Stat C section" was all I needed to hear. I had not been asleep for more than 30 minutes when the phone startled me awake. Instinctively I put on my glasses and glanced quickly at the red digital numbers flashing 12:01 AM. Since I always slept in my scrubs when on call at the hospital, it took only seconds to slip my bare feet into my wooden clogs stained with four years of brown antiseptic Betadine solution, blood, amniotic fluid, meconium, and any other female body fluid that comes from a human being. The soft, smooth wood of the inside of the clogs clung perfectly to my feet and toes, and tempered with years of these fluids, immediately grounded me.

I had never met the woman who was on the gurney being pushed into the delivery suite where the C- section would occur. One quick glance around and I could see the IV fluids running, nasal oxygen flowing, and my young female intern on her knees, on the gurney between the patient's legs in the position she had been taught for a prolapsed umbilical cord causing fetal distress – her arm high up inside the vagina, in almost to the elbow, and elevating the baby's head off the cord which had prolapsed into the upper vagina. This allowed blood and oxygen to flow to the baby about to be delivered by emergency Cesarean. This was a true obstetrical emergency when seconds mattered before fetal death or irreversible brain damage occurred. The intern knew that she and the patient would be moved to the operating table with the patient as one unit, in this position between the patient's legs, and would be covered by the surgical drapes. She would not remove her arm until I told her to do so.

As Chief Obstetrical resident on call that night, I was in charge and would be doing the emergency surgery. My mission was to have a healthy mother and baby, and to make sure everyone was doing the tasks they had been trained to do in this emergency. There was no other option, as often is the case when dealing with Mother Nature gone awry. The nurse anesthetist was monitoring the IV line and oxygen while drawing into syringes the medications needed to administer general anesthesia, and placing a heart monitor and pulse oximeter. The scrub nurse put on her surgical gown and opened the sterile instrument trays and drapes. The two circulating nurses poured sterile fluids, recorded notes and times, and did whatever anyone else asked them to do, including making sure the pediatric resident was on her way to the operating room to care for the newborn the moment birth occurred. Antiseptic brown Betadine solution had been poured on the mother's abdomen. I always loved the way it glistened on a scrubbed belly right before I was to cut it open. It was like a medical symphony happening before my eyes, yet barely open, unblinking, and basically unable to see because my glasses had fogged up due to the rapid temperature change from the on call room to the frigid operating room.

Always cold, on this night the tiled walls of the operating room were particularly frigid. The outside temperature in downtown Philadelphia at midnight in January, with snow falling, was in single digits. As I finished a 30 second scrub, I could see through the one outside window from the third floor onto Spruce street, illuminated by one yellow street light. It was mostly black outside, with snowflakes falling, the window frosted, which told me the inside room temperature was something above single digits. I glanced at the operating room clock that now read 12:03 AM. Two minutes earlier I had been dreaming of snow skiing in the Rockies somewhere. It felt like I almost got my wish!

I did my best to reassure the patient that she and the baby were going to be fine, perhaps hard for her to accept from a guy she had never met, laying there with someone's arm inside her vagina, and all the hustle and bustle surrounding her. Everyone had already explained to her what was about to happen before I showed up on the scene, so a calming presence from me was the best thing I could offer her at that moment. For some strange reason, despite the fact we had never met and I was about to put a surgical knife into her abdomen, she was remarkably calm and composed, and seemed to trust me, or so I thought. At this point, the only part of her body I could see was a small rectangle between the blue surgical drapes, exposing the belly button down to the pubic bone. Her face was now behind the anesthesia screen. And of course she had company under the drapes between her legs, my intern, who was now reporting to me that the umbilical cord between her fingers was pulsatile, although weakly so. Time continued to be of the essence. The nurse anesthetist had sedated the patient and was now intubating her. Everyone was quiet and still at this moment. I stood waiting and realized I was the only male in the room, an increasingly more common occurrence. "GO", I heard, as the intubation was completed.

I put out my right hand and without a word a scalpel appeared in it, slapped in place against my rubber gloves by the scrub nurse. With just the right amount of pressure so as not to enter the abdominal cavity and uterus, but enough to cut into the abdominal wall midline through skin, fat, fascia and muscle with one swipe of the hand, bleeders squirting all over the place and hitting the one small area of my glasses not already fogged over, the surgery began. Next I took scissors and opened the abdominal cavity carefully so as not to injure bowel or bladder, dropped the bladder out of my way with the scissors, and cut into the uterus until I saw the baby's face. I then placed my fingers into the uterus, spread the uterine incision open just so far as to give me enough room to get the baby out but not so far as to tear the uterine arteries, a potential disaster should it occur. I slipped my hand under the baby's head, elevated it onto the abdominal wall, suctioned out the mouth, clamped the cord, and handed him to the pediatrician who was now in the room. Another birthday party, one of maybe 10,000 I have attended in my lifetime. No wonder my own birthdays were always anticlimactic.

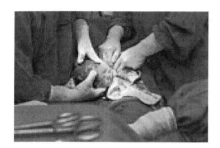

I took a moment to let the circulating nurse take off my glasses and clean the blood off them. It was instinctive on her part without me even asking. She just figured it might be a good idea if I could see before putting the patient back together.

Now there were two guys in the room! He was blinking, which seemed like such a good idea to me that I decided to do the same thing, perhaps the first blink in the last five minutes since awakening.   The operating room clock read 12:06 AM. After removing the placenta, the only thing I saw inside the uterus was the poor intern's gloved hand, which I shook as I told her she did a great job. One of the weird things we do as obstetricians, one hand of hers through the vagina into the now empty uterus, the other was mine through the abdomen and into the uterus. A little encouragement from the chief resident to the intern was always in order! She removed herself carefully from under the drapes, and went back to work on the labor and delivery deck. Her sleepless night was only beginning. Hopefully mine was about to end shortly.

Sometimes rank in the world of white -coated

doctors counts for something. As an intern, her polyester white coat was waist length short. As a Chief Resident, I got to wear mine down to my knees. And my senior faculty mentors wore thick starched white cloth coats almost down to their ankles. Seniority in a teaching hospital was everything. I got to sleep again, and she didn't. Four more years and she would be in my shoes. I suspect hers would look like mine did at this point.

Somewhere around 1 AM I was back in the on call room, snuggling under the covers, my blood stained scrubs still on, too tired to change them right now. That could wait. Sleep was more precious. I had a long day ahead with "Morning Report" awaiting presentation to our Chief of Service, several teaching clinics, more scheduled surgeries, and who knew what else Mother Nature might bring my way as the day dawned.

Falling asleep didn't always come easily with

adrenaline circulating in my system, something that would get easier to master over the years, although staying asleep for more than a few hours became a lifelong struggle and fact of life for me, as it is for many obstetricians. Random thoughts would enter my mind as I lay under the covers in the darkened room. Winter snow skiing, summer body surfing in the Atlantic City waves, weekend racquetball games, even challenging Franz Klammer to a downhill race for the Gold. Mother Nature in its many forms seemed to be the central theme, including the challenge, the mastery, the failures, but always 'The Challenge' of doing it well and correctly. I was frequently on the edge. It wasn't about winning. It was more about the effort and recognizing my own limitations, something central to being able to practice medicine well. The two were intimately and inextricably related for me. Not having any idea at any given moment as an Obstetrician what Mother Nature had in store for me was just part of life as an obstetrician. One always had to be alert, ready, sober, and awake even when sleeping. Thus the inception of what was to become a lifelong sleep disorder, an occupational hazard for me, and probably most other OB-Gyn physicians, something with which I have struggled for decades.

When I arrived in Phoenix to join my two partners, night call changed again. There were only three of us, so when we were all in town, it was an every third night every third weekend rotation. The only problem for me was as their newest junior associate and employee, and the proverbial low man on the totem pole, they were away a lot more than I was. But I was happy since I could now sleep at home rather than in the hospital. I lived close enough to the hospital that I could easily drive back and forth even multiple times during the night if necessary. Many times when someone was in labor, it was just easier to sleep at the hospital in the on call room provided. I would let the nurses know when to awaken me. They always obliged, even sooner if the situation warranted. I could slip in and out from bed at home often without my wife knowing I had left and returned, although as time wore on she got more sensitive to my comings and goings. There were times when I would be the only car on the road in the middle of the night. After a delivery was over, if all was quiet, I would speed home to catch a few winks before the day began.

Speeding was a nemesis for me. One early Sunday morning I was simply driving too fast on my way to the hospital to examine a patient in early labor. There was no particular rush on my part. But I got pulled over by a cop. I explained I was an obstetrician on my way to deliver a baby and needed to get to the hospital right away. He asked which hospital, asked for the patient's name (which of course would be a HIPPA violation had HIPPA existed then), and proceeded to follow me to the hospital parking lot, then into the labor suite and asked to see the patient's chart with her name on it. I was kind of surprised he didn't ask to examine the patient too, but that was where I had it all over him. I got off. Another time it was 2 or 3 AM and I was on my way home in my bloody scrubs after a difficult delivery. I was stopped for speeding about three blocks from my home. The officer came up to the car, took one look at me in my scrubs with fresh blood on them, and said: 'You been drinkin'? I felt like asking him if he had been drinking, but I kept quiet. I said, " No, I been deliverin' babies". No other word exchanged other than " Here is your ticket". I am not sure where he thought the blood came from, but that didn't seem to bother him.

A weekend on call in private practice meant do what you can do by yourself and only call your partners if absolutely necessary. Simply put, it was your weekend and yours alone. Occasionally we would need each other for one thing or another, but I tried my best never to call for help. My personal record was 8 deliveries in one weekend that essentially meant someone or other was contracting the whole weekend. No sooner was I putting in the last stitch for what I thought was the last delivery at 3 AM, dreaming of going home for a few hours of sleep, than I heard in the labor suite: " Hey doc, guess what, I am in labor and they told me to come right to the hospital". Such was the life of a busy OB GYN physician.

Night call became harder as I got older. Constant sleep disruption led to a worsening sleep disorder. Fortunately I learned to function with very little sleep. I could fall asleep fairly easily because I was exhausted but staying asleep became a problem probably because of the constant phone calls night after night and trips back and forth from bed to hospital. I often would recall an experiment I learned about in psychology class in college. A rat had been placed on a large cork in a tub of water. The investigator would wait until the rat was asleep then knock it off the cork into the tub of water, awakening the rat, to again place it back onto the cork and repeat this over and over again every time the rat fell asleep. Eventually the rat became psychotic, whatever a psychotic rat looked like. It seemed only a matter of time before this was to happen to me.

One night of many I awakened my wife mid night for a 'romp in the hay'. She never particularly liked the mid evening forays but then with three kids, my crazy nights, exhaustion, it had to happen when I was awake so I gently awakened her. Once she got her motor going we were usually ok. Our motors were going pretty strong when the phone rang around 2:30 AM or so. Usually it was the answering service paging me but this night it was a direct call from the Labor and Delivery nurse. "We need you now" she said. 'I am coming, I am coming, right now", I breathlessly responded. I do believe the irony went over her head.

Another night I was awakened in mid night by one of the Pediatricians to whom we referred all our babies. It was usually me needing his services in the middle of the night and not the other way around, which is why I suppose he didn't mind awakening me. He explained to me that he and his wife had sex earlier in the evening. I congratulated him and asked if he was always going to call me when that happened, and privately wondered why this was the first call. After all what else could I say in the middle of the night? Evidently she couldn't get her diaphragm out. I explained to him it was supposed to stay in for several hours anyhow, then I asked if he wanted me to come over to take it out at 2 AM. He said "No thanks!" Then I said, " John, you are a physician. Put your damn fingers inside and pull it out. There is nothing in there you are going to hurt, and nothing in there that is going to hurt you!"

Nightlife also meant social life for us. Everything of course depended on my on call schedule. We rarely wanted to, or could go out when I was on call. If we did, the night often got interrupted and my wife would have to find a ride home with someone else if I left to attend someone in labor. Worse still, if we were at a wedding, a large hospital function, or a Bar Mitzvah, as my wife says, I was often in a corner with women lined up who wanted to tell me something or other, or worse yet about their own labor experience. Alcohol seemed inclined to make that happen. So we only went to big functions out of necessity, and preferred to dine out alone, or go to a movie or small parties with friends.

Nightlife was just a continuum of day life as an obstetrician. Nothing changed that much except there were no office hours, and I could be at home with my family until the phone rang. I became adept at taking naps whenever possible, my dog Max always at my bedside napping with me. We did our best to always have family dinner together, and I did my best to always give my kids their nighttime baths and read them a story before bedtime. Not infrequently, when my daughter was little, I would fall asleep in her bed while reading night time stories to her— "Good night Moon", with the music box on. She would tip toe out to my wife and say: "Mommy, shhhh! Daddy is asleep in my bed and I want him to sleep there tonight. Don't wake him up." Invariably I would awaken a few minutes later since I couldn't stay asleep anyhow. But it was cute!

Chapter 6   Operating Room

My first surgical experience was as a second year medical student during my first OB GYN rotation at Reading Hospital. My mentor was a most interesting guy in many respects. One of the things most of us liked about him was that he let us do almost everything even though we had no idea what we were doing since we were only medical students. But he had a tremendous amount of confidence in himself, and even though he let us operate, he was always by our side, always attentive, and always teaching. For a second year medical student, it was not only nerve wracking but also quite amazing. I would not have been comfortable doing that myself for a second year medical student. There were three of us on the rotation at one time. One was a woman in my class who was short, maybe half my size, and smart as a whip. He was teaching us

how to do laparoscopic surgery, putting a
telescope into the abdominal cavity through
which one looked, made diagnoses, and then
performed surgeries. He showed us how to put
in the abdominal trocar, a sharp instrument that
required controlled blunt force to put in, after
which the sharp part is removed, a sheath left in
place, and the blunt laparoscope inserted
through the sheath. The dangerous part was
insertion of the sharp trocar since it was done
without being able to see into the abdomen at
that point. Knowledge of anatomy was critical.
He outlined the anatomy for us and was careful
to show us proper technique. After observing
several cases, he let us place the trocar ourselves.
Of course the patients were anesthetized with
legs up in stirrups. I grasped the trocar as
shown, and inserted it as shown without
problems. I was surprised at how much force
one had to use to get it through the abdominal
wall, sharp as the trocar was. The next case my
female compatriot was up. Because of her short
stature she had to stand on a stool to get in the
proper position. She then pushed with all her

might but the trocar did not go into the abdomen. She tried a second time with even more force, and it plunged way too far and fast into the abdomen and impaled the bony sacrum where it was stuck. He extracted the trocar, which was not the problem. The question was had it also damaged blood vessels or perforated bowel on the way in. Fortunately for the patient, and for all of us, it had not. She narrowly missed all vital structures and blood vessels. I never have seen a trocar impaled in the sacrum before or since! Thank goodness.

Learning operating room sterile technique was not as easy as one might expect. During another second year surgical rotation at Atlantic City Hospital, the very first thing we had to learn was how to scrub at the sink, then make it past the operating room door without touching anything, how to hold our hands so dirty water from the elbows wouldn't drip on clean hands, how to ask for and receive a sterile towel to dry our hands, then how to get into the surgical gown and gloves without contaminating anything or anyone on the scrub table, and finally how not to contaminate the surgeon when standing at the table. If one watches an experienced surgeon do it, it is much like a well-performed symphony. Watching a medical student do it is only a bit funnier than watching a medical show on TV where they have no concept of what to do with a surgical mask or at a scrub sink. The first time I tried, I never made it to the surgical table. The scrub nurse kept sending me back over and over again so that by the time I got it right, the case was over. Humbled once again. But eventually I got the hang of it and once down pat, it was like rote.

Blood and I got along just fine. Some people are squeamish at the sight of blood. Not me. Red oxygenated blood is actually a beautiful color. But I have seen grown men, husbands of Cesarean section patients who wanted to be in the operating room at delivery, literally hit the anesthesia machine with their heads as they were on their way down to the floor. Then the people in the operating room have to take care of the husband rather than the person on the operating table, never a good thing. For the uninitiated, the amount of blood admixed with amniotic fluid at the time of a Cesarean section can appear huge. Even for the initiated or about to be initiated it can at times be overwhelming. When I was a second year resident performing a Cesarean section with a newly minted intern, he got nauseous and faint in the operating room, never a good thing for a brand new intern who is under the microscope anyhow.

There was always the unexpected to deal with in medicine that could occur at any time or place, day or night. One day when on the gynecology service as a third year resident I was in the midst of a particularly difficult abdominal hysterectomy. There was considerable bleeding in a deep abdominal hole with less than optimal visualization, blood welling up from below and obscuring my view of the surgical anatomy. The scrub nurse took off her gloves and began to leave the room. I was stunned and asked her where she was going.

'Hon", she said in her thickest Philadelphia accent, "it is three o'clock and my shift is over."

"Where is your replacement?" I responded because clearly there wasn't anyone else scrubbing and there wasn't going to be.

"You have all the instruments you need, the needles and sutures are there, and you can arm everything yourself", she responded with some arrogance.

I said: "If I were the chief of neurosurgery you wouldn't be doing this."

"Hon " she said, "you are not the Chief of Neurosurgery".

Neither was I a world-renowned infertility specialist as was one of my Professors during residency. He was published, lectured all over the world, pontificated here there and everywhere, and had patients come from everywhere for his world renowned surgical expertise. The only problem was that the infertility specialist insisted that only third year, and when possible always a Chief resident, assist him at surgery. In reality we would do the surgery and he would assist. He was inept at the operating table. He was no longer capable of doing this delicate surgery with the precision it required. It was a quiet deception that was ongoing, and I didn't like any part of it. As a third year resident, when I had a chief tell me to assist, I had no choice. But as a chief resident, I never assisted him myself, especially since he was the only surgeon I have ever scrubbed with who actually cut me with a scalpel. I always gave the cases to third year residents.

As the attending surgeon in private practice, I never felt more comfortable and secure than in an operating room. It was for me a sanctuary in many respects. Surgery was often the highlight of my day. I enjoyed the satisfaction it gave to both the patient and me when it was done well with the proper indications. But anything could go wrong on any given case, so it was imperative to never put a patient in the operating room unless the surgery was indicated, and all more conservative methods of treating the condition had either been offered and rejected, or offered and tried and then failed. There was nothing worse than having a complication at surgery on a patient who didn't have to be on the table. So I never put anyone on that table unless they really had to be there. For me, when the case began, the OR door was shut, nothing on the outside world could interfere. People who called and needed me when I was in surgery had notes left on the outside of the door for me to answer when the case was over. Whatever else might be going on in my office or elsewhere in the hospital had to wait, because rarely could one leave a case in the middle to attend someone else, unless there was no choice. There were a few times when in the middle of a case, a patient would come in labor and deliver precipitously, and there was for one reason or another no one else available. On those rare occasions I would scrub out, do the delivery, then come back to the OR and finish the case, but only left if the patient was stable. The operating room was truly as the British called it, the Theater. But it was my theater, and I felt very comfortable on the stage with the bright lights on. It was a refuge from the outside world, and for me, calming.

Theater takes on different meanings depending on the day. In the midst of a difficult case one day, the OR phone rang in my room. The circulating nurse answered the call. My wife had been put through to the OR. She was with our three small kids at K Mart and locked the car keys inside the car. Attention K Mart shoppers! I had one of my office employees come down to the OR to get my keys, take them to her, and solve the emergency!

Unexpected disasters would occasionally occur. One Labor Day weekend a married, fairly young four-month pregnant patient came in with an acute abdomen. The workup indicated a ruptured large ovarian cyst with a viable intact intrauterine pregnancy. Surgery was indicated not only because of the pain, but because she was bleeding into her abdomen. When I opened her up I found a large, aggressive ruptured ovarian cancer. I removed the ovary and put out a call to the gynecologic oncologic surgeon who fortunately was available and near by the hospital on this holiday weekend. He came in; we discussed the case, and determined that her best chance for survival was to remove the pregnant uterus and other ovary then and there. We both left the operating room with her asleep and on the table to discuss the case with her husband in the waiting room, who gave us permission to do the definitive surgery. Of course it ended the pregnancy and her fertility, but there really was no choice involved. Her life was at stake. Unfortunately she died the same week her baby was due to have been born, a mere five months later. What a most unfortunate tragedy.

A ruptured pregnant uterus in a woman who is in labor is also a surgical emergency and requires immediate surgery to save the baby's life, and the mother's. It is a difficult but urgent diagnosis to make and happened to one of my patients in labor. Roughly one fifth of the maternal blood supply flows to the uterus every minute. Theoretically, in five minutes a patient can bleed to death. She was rushed to the operating room with little time for explanation to her panic stricken husband, but time was of the essence. I opened her abdomen and indeed the uterus was ruptured with the baby floating free in the abdomen. The baby was delivered quickly and did well, but the uterine rupture was so extensive that the bleeding could only be controlled by an emergency hysterectomy, a difficult and bloody operation on a full term pregnant woman, but life saving. I was working quickly, instruments and sponges were flying, and appropriate care was taken to make sure all went well, which it did. Considering it was the middle of the night, everyone performed admirably and the whole team was to be commended. As I was closing the abdominal wall and the nurses were performing the instrument and sponge counts, they determined that a surgical forceps was missing. So we moved the patient while still anesthetized and unconscious to see if it was under the drapes or behind the patient. It was not. I called in the x-ray tech to take a stat film with the patient on the table. Bright as day it lit up – inside the patient. So I had to open her up again to retrieve it. Once again, everyone was to be commended for performing their respective jobs correctly, in this case instrument counting by the nurses, during an emergency surgery. Had the scrub and circulating nurses not done things correctly, at some point an additional surgery and anesthetic would have been necessary when the instrument was found and caused problems, perhaps months later. So I went out to the waiting room to talk to the still panicked husband with a good news/bad news scenario. His baby was alive and well, as was his wife, who had to undergo an emergency hysterectomy. No more children for them, which neither of them cared about since this was their sixth. And then I slipped in the part about the forceps, a mere blip on the screen at that point. He didn't blink an eye. Honesty pays. A malpractice suit avoided.

There is an old adage that one should not operate on family members. There is nothing illegal about it, nor is it unethical, nor would I recommend it for most people. But my wife chose to become a patient of our practice for many reasons. She liked my two senior partners, and she liked the fact that I was always around should I ever be needed for anything. So when she got pregnant for the first time, she saw my partners for her obstetrical care and I kept my watchful eye on everything from the sidelines. I had always told her from the time we met that it was likely she was going to have a C-section. I was fairly good at assessing the bony pelvis, and I knew hers was small. What of course I didn't know then was the size that a future child would be. It does take a passage and a passenger to make that final determination. So as she grew with our first son, she went from about 98 pounds dry weight to over 150 pounds and wound up carrying an 8-pound boy who went two weeks beyond his due date before she went into labor. Her labor was managed by one of my partners, but it became clear progress was slow and protracted, and that no matter how much time we gave her, she was going to wind up in the operating room. After a pretty horrendous and busy day for me, not to mention how difficult her day was for her with a prolonged and protracted labor, with emergency surgeries, an office full of patients, other labors to manage, and a bad prior night on call in addition to knowing she was in labor, I managed to keep tabs on her labor until we finally decided that it was time for a Cesarean section. It was after midnight. My partner took the reigns at the table and I assisted him. He made a particularly small cosmetic incision so that when it came time to get my son out of the uterus, he struggled immensely. Then, for whatever his reasons were, he asked me to take over. I succeeded and delivered a healthy son. Subsequently I performed other procedures on her at her request, including a laparoscopy, another abdominal surgery for a large ovarian cyst, and an endometrial ablation for abnormal bleeding. She got the best care available and I enjoyed being able to provide it. Many people asked me how I could operate on my wife. For me it was a pleasure to be able to help her with her problems. For her, she was very comfortable with me doing the procedures otherwise she would not have asked. The only thing that did bother me was before the laparoscopic procedure I looked over the anesthesia screen to see her face after she was asleep, and her eyes were wide open. I asked the anesthesiologist to tape them closed. Of course, I never billed her insurance for the procedures. I tell people that one of the many differences between me and OJ is that we both cut open our wives. The difference is that I put mine back together with loving care.

One Sunday morning when I was watering my grass outside my house, I got a call from one of my partners who asked me to come in to do a hysterectomy on his wife. I knew her well, personally and socially, but she was not and had never been my patient. His mother was my patient, but not his wife. He told me she had come into the emergency room during the night with heavy bleeding and he decided she needed, and she decided she wanted, a vaginal hysterectomy, removal of the uterus through the vagina without an abdominal incision. I told him I was uncomfortable with this since she had never been my patient. I didn't know her from a medical standpoint but they were both insistent. I trusted his judgment. I knew they wouldn't have asked if they both didn't want it done and if he felt it was needed. Besides, her labs indicated she was indeed bleeding heavily. They had three children and were done with childbearing. So in I went, examined her, and decided to proceed. They would have had it no other way. The surgery went without incident. That one time she became my patient. The following day in the hospital on rounds I decided to do a medical workup to see if there had been any other underlying medical problems that could have caused the bleeding. Sure enough she was diagnosed with a rather severe thyroid disease that needed to be treated medically, undoubtedly the real reason for the abnormal bleeding. Had it been diagnosed before the surgery the procedure could likely have been avoided. I would always screen for thyroid disease in my patients having abnormal bleeding, and rarely if ever was it diagnosed. It figures that in this case that would happen. A lesson learned. I had a happy patient, a happy husband and partner, but an unhappy surgeon! My Chief of Service at Pennsylvania Hospital would have been unhappy with me, too, if I presented this case at morning rounds. One should never deviate from what one knows to be good medicine.

Chapter 7   Abortion

Skilled medical and surgical provision of abortion services is necessary, appropriate, legal, and a diminishing skill which needs to be preserved so that women's health care will continue to be top notch without stepping backwards into the dark ages from which it emerged almost 40 years ago. I can't honestly say that when I was considering medicine I gave any thought to whether or not I would be involved with abortion services, nor did I seek it out or proselytize for it. It just became part of my life and training when I chose the field of Obstetrics and Gynecology.

When in college I enrolled in an introductory philosophy course, about which I knew nothing, to broaden my horizons. Fortunately it was offered as a Pass/Fail course rather than for a grade. We had to write papers about all kinds of subjects. I just couldn't get my head around how to write a philosophy paper, unlike papers I had to write for other courses in college. One of the assignments was about the topic of 'Abortion', which I delved into deeply. It was really my first exposure to the topic and the first time I had given it any thought. In 1968 it was pre Roe versus Wade and hotly discussed. Abortion was still illegal, yet women were finding ways to have them performed without regard to their own health. I couldn't possibly take any other position than pro choice supporting abortion. There was just no other way for me to see the issue. I wrote a strong pro-choice abortion paper. For me a woman's rights to control her own body superseded anything else no matter what the circumstances of the pregnancy. It was her body and she could do with it whatever God given right she chose to do with it, as could I with mine. It was as simple as that. There seemed to me nothing more desirable, sweet, and pleasant than a wanted pregnancy, and from the viewpoint of a sociology and psychology student, nothing worse than an unwanted/unplanned pregnancy for the fetus, the mother, the family, or society at large. It seemed black and white to me. I got my first and only red "F" on a paper I had written in college. Not so much for the stand I had taken and supported, but for the fact that I took a stand at all and refused to see the merits, pros and cons, of the other side. Fortunately, I passed the course but this solitary event played a large part in shaping my early views about women, society, reproductive and individual rights and choice.

During one evening shift in the emergency room as a second year medical student in Center City Philadelphia, a young 13-year old African American girl was brought in with an acute abdomen, hemorrhaging from the vagina with fetal tissue visible at the cervix, the opening to the uterus. It was 1973, and Roe versus Wade had just been passed by the Supreme Court with a 7-2 decision giving a woman the right to privacy under the due process clause of the 14th Amendment of the constitution. This extended the right to a woman to have an abortion until the age of fetal viability. It overturned and voided a Texas state law of criminal abortion.

For this young girl in front of me the law was too little and too late. It was never clear what the circumstances were that led her to a back alley in North Philadelphia, where some uncaring and untrained profiteer put a coat hanger inside her cervix and uterus to cause the abortion. She was left septic, hemorrhaging, with a perforated uterus and ruptured intestines. Septic shock is never a good thing to have or to watch. Her medical team, of which I was just a non-participant observer at the time, struggled for days to keep her alive. It was an eye opener for me - an emergency hysterectomy, removal of tubes and ovaries, bowel repair, IV antibiotics, days in the ICU before her senseless death at the age of 13 from septic shock. Almost everything I had studied and learned as a sociology major in four years of college was embodied in this one destitute young woman in front of me for days; poverty, illiteracy, family dysfunction, lack of contraception and access to good health care, sexual abuse, social ills, profiteering, and abortion. All of society's terrible problems were brought to bear on this one young woman. It was a horrible thing to see and watch, and left an indelible impression on me that I carry with me to this day. It was at that moment that my thoughts about caring for women began to crystallize. Hopefully as the years went by, Roe V Wade would bring this all to an end. In my mind the Supreme Court got it right then. No Court since then has seen fit to overturn this momentous decision and hopefully none ever will. "Settled law" is the term used now, and settled it should be no matter who sits on the Supreme Court now or in the future. To overturn this law will send our country and our women back into the Dark Ages.

During my second year of training at Pennsylvania Hospital I spent three months in what was called a Family Planning Rotation, where we discussed contraceptive options with patients, performed permanent sterilization in the form of tubal ligations on those women who no longer desired fertility, and performed pregnancy terminations on women who requested the procedure. During the day we attended the Family Planning clinic, prescribed birth control, placed IUD's, fit diaphragms, discussed permanent sterilizations and scheduled and performed tubal ligations.

We also learned the ins and outs of surgical abortion training, an integral part of our training program. Since Roe V Wade was now the law of the land, abortion training was critically important to learn how to size an early pregnant uterus, what various kinds of procedures we needed to learn and perform depending on gestational age, and how to manage and deal with potential complications. Anyone could have opted out of this training if they had objections but in our program no one did while I was there. Early abortions up to 12 weeks, the first trimester, were handled in the outpatient surgical suite under a brief general anesthetic and a procedure called a suction D and C. Second trimester abortions were done by intra amniotic prostaglandin induction of labor that required learning how to perform amniocenteses, placement of a needle and catheter into the pregnant uterus through the abdomen, instilling a medication into the uterus to cause labor and subsequent delivery of a stillborn premature fetus. For me it was all part and parcel of caring for women. There was no judgment as to circumstances that brought these patients to us. But at their request, and within the guidelines of the law, we learned the skill of providing a safe, simple service that preserved their fertility for later years when the women were ready to have children. All the women followed up with us in the Family Planning clinic. It was as it should be to guarantee women good health and reproductive care and rights. There were no advertising of services, no protests, and no mishaps and loss of fertility and life as I had experienced a few years earlier in the Hahnemann emergency department.

First trimester pregnancy terminations were already a routine part of our practice in Phoenix when I arrived. One of my partners had been medical director of Planned Parenthood during his first year in Arizona. He established a referral network for pregnancy terminations in the city. Our group was one of a number of providers for early pregnancy terminations. In those days Planned Parenthood did the counseling, the testing, and made the referrals. Over subsequent years they eventually hired physicians in house to do the procedures and stopped referrals to the community physicians, a business decision with which I disagreed. It seemed to me that money became more of a motivating factor for the organization rather than counseling which had been their charter. But so be it. That was their decision.

My partners chose long before I arrived to do only first trimester pregnancy terminations that were performed in the office under a local anesthetic and sedation early in the morning before regular office hours. This was a progressive move for me since in training all the procedures I had performed were accomplished under a general anesthetic in outpatient surgery. So I quickly had to develop in office skills at sedation and local anesthesia, and operating on and talking to patients who were awake. It was a valuable skill to have learned quickly in private practice that came to serve me well for the future, as well as lessen risk for the patient. There was no advertising for these procedures. There were no protests outside the office. Patient privacy, protection, and comfort were important to us. We gave each patient the time, counseling and comfort needed to make sure of her decision without the stress of people carrying placards and harassment. We followed up with the patient three weeks later with a routine exam, a pregnancy test to make sure it was negative, and contraceptive counseling. Many of these forever-grateful women became life long patients of the practice and we became their obstetricians over the years.

Not long after my arrival in Arizona, Senator Barry Goldwater and his wife sponsored a party at his home in Paradise Valley, Arizona to benefit Planned Parenthood. A six term US Senator and former Republican Presidential candidate against Lyndon Johnson in 1964, he was the true father of Republican conservatism and a Libertarian. He always frankly spoke his mind. Although I rarely agreed with what he said politically I admired him for his honesty and patriotism, in short supply nowadays. So I chose to go to his home. As most folks did not know and as today's conservative and Tea Party Republican's would vilify him for, he and his wife Peggy were strong supporters of

Planned Parenthood, a woman's Right to Choose, and keeping "the damn government out of people's bedrooms" as the Senator so aptly put it. This was consistent with his Libertarian and personal philosophy. One reason he lost the Presidential election was because he did speak his mind and not everyone liked what they heard, but he was true to his beliefs and honest which I greatly respected. Today's Republicans would do well to read their history books.

So three months into Arizona I found myself inside Senator Goldwater's beautiful home on a mountaintop overlooking the city. His wife spoke and they were gracious hosts. We had free roam of his house so my wife and I poked around. We were strolling, cocktail in hand down a long hallway when the Senator appeared from inside a room. He introduced himself and asked us if we would like to see something special. He took us into his Gun Room lined with cabinets filled with rifles and guns of all sorts. He pulled out a ladder, climbed it (he wasn't a young man then), opened a cabinet, took down a rifle from the top cabinet and put it in my hands. I was polite, non-gun supporter that I was. After all I was in his home. There wasn't much I could do but take it. He asked me if I knew what I was holding. Other than ' a rifle' there wasn't much else I could say. He proceeded to explain to us that it was the best rifle ever made, one used by the 'Red Chinese" as he called them, in the early 1900's. And so my introduction to Arizona continued.

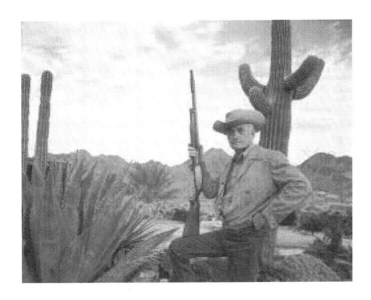

One of the hospital committees on which I sat was Credentials. This committee reviewed and gave hospital privileges to new staff applicants. One monthly meeting there was an application from an OB GYN doctor, well trained, an Army veteran, applying for staff privileges. His credentials were in order and there was no reason to deny him admitting privileges. The only concern for me was his letterhead on normal size stationary with his name in such large bold face print that it consumed about 2/3 of the page. I had never quite seen professional stationary like that before and it raised a red flag for me. As it turned out he performed late second and even early third trimester abortions. He was one of the only physicians in the State of Arizona who did so. He pushed the limits at all ends and wasn't one of my favorite people on earth. He was all over the news in the subsequent months. There were always protesters in front of his office. He loved the attention. One day I saw him in the operating theater changing room, bullet vest on and holstered pistol under his arm. This was his chosen life. Years later as I followed his career, he was accused and convicted of sexual molestation of a patient and wound up in State prison. For some reason I wasn't all that surprised. Fortunately, he was a unique person.

As to the women who sought abortion, there was truly nothing they had in common other than they had an unwanted, unplanned pregnancy. They came from all walks of life; the rich and the poor; the black and the white; the professional and the non- professional; the religious and the agnostic; the pro choice, and the Right to Lifers. Yes, it was interesting to see some folks come off the picket line for the service we provided when it affected them. Whatever stereotypes there are out there about women who seek abortion should be forgotten. Pregnancy is a momentous decision in anyone's life, whether an unwanted or wanted pregnancy. It should not be forced on anyone for any reason whatsoever, for there are truly few things in life that are so life altering. Thus to legislate against a woman's right to choose is society forcing a woman to do something that she may not want nor be able to afford financially or emotionally, and worse may be ill prepared to handle. Bringing a child into this world to either a set of parents, or a single parent, through coercion is no way to begin a life. It will not bode well for the unborn individual. I give the utmost respect to those women who are able to have enough foresight and courage to make this difficult decision. No one but them, in consultation with their health care provider, their families, and their significant others should be interfering with an individual's right to make this decision. Senator Goldwater was able to see that, and so should everyone else from the conservative side of politics that think they know what is best for a woman and seek to legislate their beliefs into a part of life where legislation does not belong. The Supreme Court got it right when it said we are all entitled to the right of privacy under the constitution. For any future providers of women's services, it should be known that this is a skill, like any other medical skill, that should continue to be taught, learned, and provided with privacy and dignity for everyone concerned.

Chapter 8 Business of Medicine

Medicine is an art. It is medical science. And it is a business.

When I first started medical school, I really hadn't given that any thought. I just assumed I would manage to make a living somehow. One of the unique things Hahnemann did with us as freshman medical students was early on require us to spend an evening a week in a family medicine or primary care practice somewhere in Philadelphia that they had prearranged for us. We were to do nothing other than sit and observe.

I was sent into the heart of Italian South Philadelphia to the home office of a general practitioner. One could almost taste the Philly cheese steaks from across the street, and only imagine the fresh pasta with gravy followed by a cannoli cooking in the row home kitchens next to his.

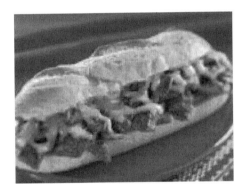

(Cheese steaks – the best!)

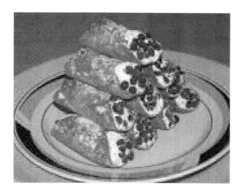

(Good Cannoli's)

He had a small waiting room and a large office
with an even larger desk behind which he sat,
with me off to the side in a chair saying nothing
and observing everything. I was wide eyed. He
did it all himself without a nurse. The patients
were all his friends and neighbors, would sit in
front of his desk, he would hug them, make small
talk and chat, take their blood pressures, find out
what was new in their lives, and then finally talk a
little medicine with them. Sometimes, but not
always, he would even examine them. When all
was said and done, they would get up and give

him a $20 bill. He reached into his pants pocket and pulled out a large green wad of cash. He gave them change to one degree or another. This was my introduction to the business of medicine. I decided then and there that I was never going to talk to patients about money. There had to be some better way. What it was I didn't know, but I was going to figure it out.

As an intern and resident, I was paid a salary by the hospital. It was meager but combined with my wife's wages we made about $30,000 per year between us by the end of my fourth year of residency. Thanks to my parents I had no debt, unlike many medical students today. Since we spent $1000 /month on our apartment, it left us enough for food, an occasional movie and cheap wine, and a few meals out. Nothing left to save. We both walked to work, easy to do in the city. When we left Philly to go to Phoenix, I had signed a three year contract with increasing salaries guaranteed as long as they liked me, the practice continued to grow, and they wanted me to continue to work. Our needs were meager, were met and afforded us enough to start a family.

One of my partners controlled the purse strings when I was an employee. I had no idea how the business of medicine worked, the process of medical insurance, managed care, payroll, or anything to do with money other than when to expect my paycheck, and how to correctly mark for the billing office whatever procedures I did so that the practice could somehow bill and collect for my services performed. As an employee it was best this way anyhow, since I had my medical practice to build and concentrate on, the family medicine residents to teach and mentor, and my oral Board examinations for certification for which to prepare. I also had a baby on the way.

After three years as an employee, I was given the option of buying shares of the medical corporation and becoming an equal share holder, which entitled me to equal salary as my other two partners minus the cost of the buy in. We did not work on a productivity basis. It was assumed we would all work equally hard, and bring in equally as much money, so we all got an equal salary. This was the "corporate culture" I bought into, and I had no problem with it. The only difference between us was I got less vacation than my partners, but over time that equalized too. I chose to go to the bank and borrow the cost of the buy in so that I could immediately make the same salary as my partners. My wife and I had never borrowed so much money before. Nor had we ever had that kind of salary. When it came time for the banker to come to have us sign the papers, it was a short time after I had rather seriously injured my back during a fall from a hammock onto a brick patio (my fault but we needn't go there). I had been bedridden on narcotics for two weeks and I could barely walk. My wife, two small kids and I were holed up at a local hotel with a special weekend deal and a nice pool for the weekend, a nice place to recover. So the banker nicely enough came to the hotel to have us sign the papers. He knew nothing about my back. Perhaps he found it strange that I didn't stand when he came in the room, and remained seated in the chair the whole time. I wasn't about to let him know that I couldn't walk, for if he did, he probably never would have given me the loan.

Over time, when I became a partner in a thriving business, I learned more and more about the business of medicine. One of my partners ran the whole business from his office, and the other had nothing to do with the business side but was more entrepreneurial. Everyone contributed in his own way. But it was an old fashioned way, though successful, of running a modern medical business, probably the same way his Dad had run his medical office years earlier in Philadelphia. No computers, checks written by hand, invoices paid by hand written checks, scheduling done with a pencil in a large schedule book, etc. Medicine in general, and

Phoenix in particular, was changing drastically. The 'Golden era' of medicine had ended. I was only slightly privy to catching the tail of this age of medicine when I was in residency. We residents used to call some of the surgical procedures the 'blue plate special'. Exam under anesthesia, D and C, hysterectomy, salpingo-oophorectomy (removal of tubes and ovaries), lysis of adhesions, and anything else that could be listed separately, each one of which came with a separate reimbursement. The more one could list, the more one collected. That is what brought an end to the "Golden age of Medicine". Physicians ruined it for themselves. But that was the past. I had to learn the system going forward.

The payment scenario was changing dramatically. Phoenix was the epicenter of it all. There were few Mom and Pop employers, and many large companies headquartered in a rapidly expanding city. Managed care took a strong foothold in Phoenix, and over time expanded nationwide. To my former colleagues in the East

I used to say, be prepared, it is coming your way, which it did. Since there was no way to fight it, best to learn about managed care, how it worked, and how to maximize reimbursement if that were possible. That became my contribution to the business side of our practice. After countless business and managed care meetings that I attended, I came to understand that there was only one way to succeed financially in this kind of managed care and Medicaid environment. The business office needed to be computerized from top to bottom. We needed to find a way to have a high volume, low overhead practice and manage the volume professionally. In essence, we needed to run the business like an airlines. Everyone would be treated kindly and equally, no one would be refused care regardless of payment method, everyone would get the same professional service, we would do our best to get every patient into the office the day they called if at all possible (get the seats filled), we would always try to get new patients in immediately when they called (why give them the chance to go somewhere else if they needed to be seen now and were on the phone?). We joined every managed care program that was available to us and accepted whatever insurance paid for services rendered, and did whatever we needed to collect the insurance reimbursements in a timely manner. We accepted the fact that some people would sit next to each other in the waiting room, receive the same service, and some would pay more, or less, than others, a price determined not by us but by contract with the payor (the insurance company or government). No one would know. Do you know what the guy seated next to you pays when you fly? The business office managed our aged accounts receivable aggressively. We discounted our services to those who had no insurance and could only pay cash. We accepted credit cards. We used a collection agency for those patients who needed to be sent to collections, but we would still continue to see these patients.

One of my partners decided to retire at about

this point because he was ready to move on, and to some degree because he didn't like the changes in the business of medicine. So I willingly became the chief financial officer of the corporation, which pleased my other partner and allowed him to pursue his other entrepreneurial ideas, in which I also actively participated. But the business became mine to run, a challenge I gladly accepted, despite the lowest score ever seen on my college aptitude test for accounting.

We expanded our office to larger quarters to not only accommodate a rapidly enlarging patient load, but also a rapidly enlarging staff needed to deal with the patient load. We also made the decision to invest money in a state of the art computer system for the business side of the practice. This included modules that ran the scheduling, accounts receivable, billing, payroll, and accounting. In 1988 electronic medical records were still in the future. We expanded over the years from the three original partners to eventually 14 health care providers, four offices throughout the city, a total of 80 employees, and staff privileges at five hospitals, while operating from only one business office. Fortunately we had infrequent employee turnover. When I found the right employee, I asked them what they expected in salary, and would almost always find that we would match their expectations. In fact, often people asked for less than what I was willing to pay. If someone was good and felt they could do the job, we paid them what was necessary to get the job done properly. Professionalism was critical, and the staff was happy.

Our original philosophy did not change. High quality health care, personalized service to everyone regardless of financial status, and refusing no one were all high priorities. If someone called us and wanted to be seen, they were seen that day if possible. It made for a very busy life - a full time OBGYN with a large patient load, managing what I came to later find out was the largest non hospital based health care business in the State of Arizona. I had come a long way from the guy who was told never to be an accountant. I did payroll myself every two weeks on the computer in my office, I entered and paid all invoices after reviewing them to make sure they were correct, and I kept daily tabs on both collections and aged accounts receivable. I hired and fired employees when necessary, and helped recruit and interview new associates. I signed insurance contracts. It was fun, challenging, and at times stressful. It was a large responsibility.

Meeting payroll every two weeks for 80 corporate employees was a challenge but never once over the 12 years that I ran the business was it not met. Every year we would have a corporate barbecue in a local Phoenix park for all employees, their spouses and kids. One year I agreed to flip the burgers. It dawned on me as I made burgers for some 300 people that year that we were literally and figuratively feeding a lot of mouths.

I was also true to the promise that I made myself when sitting in the south Philadelphia doctor's office watching him pull that wad of cash from his pocket - that I would never personally discuss money with a patient. It was all medicine for me with the patient. If she needed something done in the way of a procedure, she went to the business office for the financial discussion and insurance questions, and if she paid cash which patients rarely did in the managed care and State Medicaid environment of Phoenix or needed a discount, my staff had advanced permission to negotiate. I was happy with the arrangement.

One year when reviewing the annual statements provided by the 'real' accountant, who had my computer generated paper trail to follow each month, one figure stuck out above all the others. Office overhead was 38% that year. Meaning the other 62% was available for the partners. This was exceptional efficiency of

which I was rightly proud for such a large
operation.

When I was finishing my residency prior to
leaving for Phoenix, one of my future partners
asked me to visit a physician in Philadelphia who
was one of the original clinical investigators
performing a new in office female sterilization
procedure under an FDA (Food And Drug
Administration) approved protocol. He told me
he, too, was going to become an investigator and
wanted me to observe and ultimately perform
the procedure with him after my arrival to
Phoenix. At the time, I knew nothing about
clinical investigation, but I was eager to learn the
new procedure. It was done by inserting a
hysteroscope through the cervix after
administration of a local anesthetic, a small fiber
optic scope through which one looks into the
interior of the uterus to view the opening of the
Fallopian tubes as they enter the uterus. Once
visualized, the Fallopian tubes had a small
catheter inserted with the silicone rubber

instilled into the tube through the catheter to block the tube and prevent conception from occurring. Most exciting about the procedure was that it had the potential to be reversed since the newly formed plug had a loop on it for retrieval.

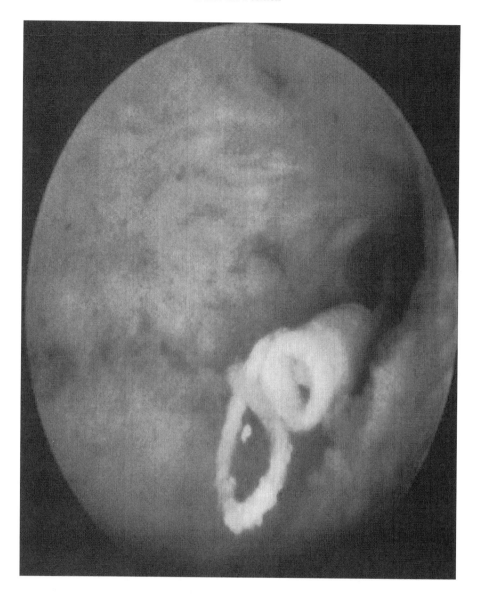

(Formed in place silicone plug with retrieval loop
resting in the tubal ostium as seen through the

hysteroscope.)

However, since the patients had been told it was permanent sterilization, the reversal was only a potential future possibility also ripe for exploration. No one knew if the tubes would actually work if the plugs were removed, or even if the plugs could be removed. Also no one yet knew exactly how effective the plugs were in preventing pregnancy. This is why the research was being done under an investigative protocol with FDA approval.

When I got to Phoenix my partner and I got involved in this procedure in a big way. It was new to me, but very exciting and cutting edge for us both. The patients paid nothing for the procedure, would come to the office over lunchtime, and 30 minutes later leave sterilized and go back to work. No major anesthesia, no major surgery, no cutting, no trauma, and sterilized with potential reversal. We were careful to only recruit women who wanted permanent sterilization since there were no guarantees either about sterilization or reversal, but such was the nature of an investigative protocol and an as yet unapproved device. The company conducting the study and owner of the patent rights paid us for successful completion of the procedure and follow up according to the protocol. Over time, we did somewhere close to 1000 of these procedures in the office and followed the patients for years, as one would have to do to determine sterilization effectiveness. We accumulated massive amounts of data that I decided to publish in the major obstetrical journals and textbooks, also an unanticipated, time consuming, but interesting venture. My partner and I travelled and lectured. We learned how to videotape the procedure for educational purposes. From a medical standpoint, it turned out to be very effective and safe. From a reversibility standpoint, it was in fact reversible with successes that we reported over time. From a safety standpoint it was indeed safe without long-term consequences.

From a financial standpoint for our practice, not just in terms of immediate financial gain but also in terms of the notoriety it brought us, it was also a success. From the standpoint of the FDA, they insisted on long term further animal studies to document safety and efficacy, and the sponsor simply ran out of money to conduct that part of the ongoing investigation. As a result, the sponsor pulled the study from the US and moved it to Europe, where the FDA did not exist, so it never got approved in the US for eventual use, an unfortunate outcome since it proved to be safe and effective.

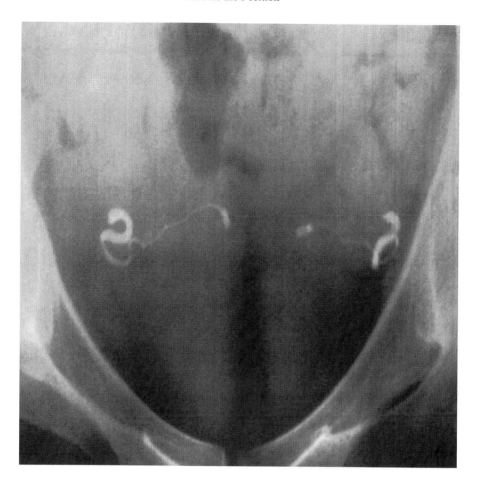

(Formed in place silicone plugs in the Fallopian tubes as seen by X-ray post procedure.)

The experience for us whetted our appetite for further clinical investigations. We were able to propel our expertise, publications, and experience into establishing Women's Health Research of Arizona. Over the ensuing years, we participated in over 35 investigative studies in the field of Obstetrics and Gynecology, testing FDA approved protocols on new medications, new contraceptives, and new medical techniques for the treatment of abnormal uterine bleeding in lieu of a hysterectomy. We were in the forefront of investigative clinical medicine testing devices not even used in teaching programs at residency programs throughout the US, so we commonly had both attending and resident visitors to our office for teaching and learning. I had little time for the management of this part of the business and was fortunate that my partner ran the research end. He enjoyed the notoriety that it brought, the travelling, and the business of making Women's Health Research profitable, which it clearly was. We got to the point where large pharmaceutical companies and device manufacturers would seek us out. New studies just began to appear for us by reputation only. I enjoyed the medical, clinical and investigative part of the work that kept us far in advance of other practices in town and on the cutting edge of new and exciting medicine. In fact, some of the more astute local practitioners got wind of what we were doing, and we had no problem with them coming to our office to observe and learn. Teaching was just part of the experience. This side venture of the practice, all self taught and conceived, satisfied our inner need for academic medicine and clinical investigation. It was fun to build from scratch, it was innovative, and it was indeed entrepreneurial.

Being on the staff of a hospital came with admitting and surgical privileges. If that is all one wanted, nothing else was required. But since my primary office was adjacent to the hospital, and this was where we planted our stake, I chose to get actively involved in hospital politics, initially as preceptor for the family medicine program, a member of the OB GYN committee, and then membership on the credentials and residency advisory committees. Eventually I was elected as chairman of the OB-GYN committee for four years. In this capacity as chairman of a department committee, I was also required to sit on the hospital executive committee. So I became intimately involved with all aspects of hospital committee work and hospital politics. There were many meetings to attend, often into the evening hours. There was no remuneration that came as a result, but a great opportunity to serve the hospital and help it grow, expand and remain successful. It also gave me the opportunity to push for my agenda to modernize both the nursery and the Labor and Delivery facilities, which were in need of expansion and modernization. During my tenure as Chairman, we created a new labor and delivery suite, new Cesarean section operating rooms designated just for OB GYN staff use apart from the general surgical suite, new post partum rooms, new on call rooms for the physicians, and a new outpatient surgery suite, all of which I was active in planning and helping to design. I actively pushed to get the nursery upgraded by the State of Arizona to a level II facility so that we could keep most sick babies in the nursery without having to transfer them, and getting neonatologists on staff. I helped establish an in house epidural service under the tutelage of nurse anesthetists supervised by anesthesiologists. Clearly obstetrical care and facilities was upgraded from when I first arrived. I was most proud of helping to get our hospital to this point. There was no financial gain to our group other than seeing the hospital more successful and welcoming to our patients, and those of the other attending physicians on staff.

From my first day of arrival in Phoenix, I was asked to be the Obstetrical and Gynecologic attending and supervising physician for the family medicine residency program at our hospital. This required me to go to their weekly OB-GYN clinic, attend their deliveries, allow them to assist and occasionally perform Cesarean sections since many of these Family Medicine residents chose to go into rural health care and needed to learn the procedure. Having just come from a high-powered residency myself, this was nothing other than just continuing what I had already been doing. More importantly, it gave me the opportunity to get to know the residents well, and vice versa. When they graduated from the program, some stayed on staff at the hospital, and they became a referral source for new patients for our practice. At some point we got the idea that we should just hire one of the residents and purchase a local family practice if and when the opportunity became available, then set up our own ancillary family medicine practice from which we could cross refer medical patients, and the medical practice could cross refer OB-GYN patients. Indeed at one point we found an interested, busy, well-respected local family physician interested in selling his practice and reducing his stress. We hired a new young resident willing to work with him and us. The practice was relocated across the hall from ours. Literally with the papers on his desk and ready to sign, the physician unfortunately died suddenly about one week before we were ready to consummate the deal. It was shocking for us all. I attended his funeral and was just simply astounded at how many friends and patients were there. After an appropriate time period, we did finally purchase the practice from his widow, and set the resident up by himself in the practice. He had fully expected to have a working partner and was a trooper the first year, after which we hired and recruited a second and third graduating resident, moved the practice to a larger location adjacent to another local hospital, and it was up and running and flourishing. We maintained and operated the business part of that practice for a number of years before selling it to the hospital. It was just a lot of work for me and I was glad to pass it off.

The business of medicine also involved the business of finding, recruiting, training, interviewing, and hiring prospective partners, then finding a way to make them busy and productive from their first day of practice. When I first joined the practice as the third physician, we were doing 12-15 deliveries per month amongst the three of us. They had plans for me to bring in new business, and to assist with their patient loads, particularly since one of the benefits of the group practice as they envisioned it was the opportunity to take time away from medicine to travel, pursue other hobbies or interests, and catch up on missing sleep. Fifteen years later we were doing 150 deliveries a month, had four flourishing offices, 14 providers, and a mixture of physicians, nurse midwives and physician assistants.

As we grew, we recruited and found new physicians who had complementary skills. Most important to us, however, was in addition to physician personalities and skills that they understood the corporate philosophy; how we practiced medicine, night call, patient sharing, group practice, vacation time, and days off. It was assumed that productivity would be equal and not become an issue. We carefully screened applicants to ensure this would not become a problem in the future and that we were compatible. The underlying theme was that salary and benefits would all equalize over time, after a period as an employee with increasing salary (now only 2 years as opposed to three when I started), a buy in as a partner would occur, financed by the practice if that was their choosing, but that one had to put in time first, be productive or at least equally so, and go to work hard from day one. We never added anyone after me unless the volume and the work were already there to support the addition. It had been a winning formula for me. We thought it would be for everyone else.

For years it was a highly successful formula. We got along well, the practice flourished, and everyone was very well paid. Not everyone had equal skills and interests, which was perfectly acceptable. Whenever possible we would self refer within the practice. For example, some folks did not want to do abortions themselves or had not been trained to do them. Not everyone enjoyed performing amniocentesis. We all did ultrasound, and had four ultrasound machines, one in each office. Not everyone wanted to be involved in clinical research. No one else had an interest running the finances of the practice or involvement in the business of medicine. Not everyone wanted to aggressively pursue new business opportunities. Everyone was just asked and expected do the work that was there, do it well without complaints, show up every day, enjoy their work and work hard.

What did become a problem over time was that not everyone worked at the same pace, and not everyone wanted to so that productivity did became an issue, as did petty jealousies. What also became a problem, though it was never visible or even discussed with me, was that not everyone enjoyed the wide diversity of patients we had in the practice. To me, a woman who needed our services should be a patient. Who she was, or where she came from, or what niche of society she came from was of no consequence to me. We were in the business of providing reproductive medicine services to women. Period. But not everyone evidently saw it that way.

As we expanded, I was asked by some of my then partners to explore the opportunity of opening a new office in the more upscale Paradise Valley section of Phoenix, which I willingly pursued. I was glad to finally see some interest in a new venture that was conceived by my younger partners even though they did not have the ability or wherewithal to get it off the ground by themselves. It took much time and energy for me to do so, finding a new office space in a brand new building adjacent to the hospital, building out the space from scratch, and furnishing it from scratch with the latest and best equipment and furnishings, lease signing, etc. It was clearly an investment for the practice, since it took funds but seemed well worth the expense. We had to recruit and reassign new office personnel. Everything that was necessary to get a brand new office up and running in a new part of town, from specula, to lights, medical equipment and ultrasound, to exam tables, computers, furniture, the whole gamut. Then further working out arrangements for night call and divesting their positions from our other offices. When all was said and done, it was a beautiful office and successful from day one.

Much to my surprise, naïve and unassuming as I was, I came to a routine partner's business meeting one day after work to face a mutiny from four 'partners'. I had spent incredible time setting them up in this new office, in addition to teaching them the ins and outs and all my experience gleaned over the years about how to run a business and make a living as an OB GYN physician in Phoenix. The long and short of it was they announced they no longer wanted to be partners. They wanted out of the practice, and they wanted the new office for themselves. I was blindsided, hurt, annoyed, angry, deceived and mostly disappointed not only in them, but also in my own lack of insight. They gave the rest of us two options. Either buy them out of the practice according to the buy sell agreement we had; or just give them the new office, furnishings, equipment, personnel and patient load, and they would be gone. I was never so disappointed with four human beings in my life. On the one hand, I guess I should have been happy that they liked, and deserved, each other as much as they did, since they had all been hand picked over the years and evidently got along quite well with each other. On the other hand, it was the most deceitful thing I had ever seen or been a part of. They had arrived in Phoenix, as did I, with not a single patient of their own or without any knowledge of how to build a practice or run one. They learned everything from those of us who preceded them, including clinical research in which they rarely participated. I suppose I was naïve and trusting, which evidently I clearly had been, because the rest of us who were being deserted knew nothing of the scheming and behind the back machinations that went on. They learned the business of medicine from us, they learned how to get what they wanted, they wanted cleaner and more upscale patients to their liking, they wanted hand picked office personnel that they recruited from our offices behind our back, they hired a lawyer, they wanted and wanted. They had been very well paid for their services over the years, despite less than equal productivity, which was clear from the accounting figures that had been kept over the years. Yet they had derived equal salaries and benefits. What dismayed and disappointed me the most was my own poor judgment in assessing their personalities. After hours of legal arguments, they got what they wanted. I was glad to see them go and get on with my life without them. Everything in life is a learning experience. Such is the business of medicine. My wife had expressed doubts from the beginning about the ringleader, but I failed to listen! If only I had trusted my wife's judgment from the beginning. She was indeed correct.

The legal definition of medical malpractice is when a physician violates what is the accepted standard of care for a physician practicing in the same state given the same or similar set of circumstances, and that the violation of standard of care directly caused the injury sustained to the patient. It does not mean that just because there is a bad outcome, i.e. a maloccurrence, that malpractice has occurred, a concept that the average layperson is not easily able to distinguish. In many cases a lawyer is unable to distinguish this difference as well. Lawyers are thus obligated to find an expert witness in the field who can advise them whether or not the standard of care was violated and caused the injury. Conversely, the defense team will also try to find an expert witness to opine the contrary, stating there either was no violation of standard of care, or that there was a violation but it did not cause the injury. This leads often to dueling witnesses in the courtroom, and the jury must decide who to believe, what other circumstances were at play, and if there should be a financial award and how much. If there is a reward, it is paid from the physician's medical malpractice insurance carrier to the injured party. Physicians are required to have malpractice insurance in most states, and most hospitals will not allow credentialing of a physician unless they show proof of malpractice insurance from the carrier. Thus physicians must purchase malpractice insurance at a hefty cost (the premium) which is determined by the insurance company, and over which the physician has no control.

The crisis is a two-fold crisis. First, the cost to the physician is enormous. At its worst when I was in active practice, the only malpractice carrier in Arizona charged OB GYN physicians and neurosurgeons the highest premiums, ours being $100,000 per year/per physician just for the right to practice medicine. If one didn't pay, one couldn't practice. It was outrageous and unacceptable, but there was no choice. The second part of the crisis was in some states where physicians did not have the financial ability to make that annual premium payment; they couldn't practice medicine and had to leave the state to practice elsewhere. This caused shortages of certain medical specialties in some states, with few options for patients who needed the medical care. Thus, the medical malpractice crisis was created.

The insurance company that hires the legal defense team clearly wants to minimize their insurance losses. Thus, at times, the insurance company will offer a settlement after a lengthy deposition process rather than go to trial to find out what in fact happened, and what the plaintiff's expert witness has to say under oath and cross examination by the defense team during the deposition. This results in a large number of medical malpractice cases pursued by patients with the remedy from the courts, if found negligent, being financial remuneration for the injured or the plaintiff. In some states, such as Arizona, the mere filing of a case also triggers a review of the facts of the case by the State Board of Medical Examiners, with the possibility of restrictions of one's license to practice medicine, or worse yet loss of license and livelihood.

My first experience with all of this was as a resident physician in Philadelphia. During the daytime I was on the GYN service, but at night when on call I needed to perform a Cesarean section on a patient who had been acutely ill with preeclampsia, a hypertensive disease of pregnancy, and worsening for days. She remained under the watchful eyes of some fellow residents who tried to get her as far into this premature pregnancy as possible to maximize the chances for the baby. They were walking a very fine line between jeopardizing maternal welfare and maximizing the fetal welfare. Preeclampsia, a potentially severe hypertensive state of pregnancy, often presented this dynamic. When I came on call that evening and met her for the first time, I quickly realized how ill she had become and decided she needed to be delivered immediately for maternal reasons, so I became the surgeon of record on the case. The surgery went without incident, the baby turned out fine, but the patient wound up in the ICU where for the next five days the obstetrical and medical team cared for her. Unfortunately the patient expired from cardiac arrest and pulmonary edema while in the ICU five days later. I had not seen her before or since the surgery since she was not on my service, but I remained the surgeon of record. When her family decided to sue, I was named in the lawsuit, as were others. It took months to get me dropped from the suit. My defense attorney successfully argued that I was one of the few people who actually did the correct thing by recognizing how sick she was and getting her delivered. I am not sure that argument helped anyone else, but it did help me. It was, however, an emotionally trying experience, not one that I was eager to ever find myself in again.

The busier and more successful our practice became in Phoenix over the years, the more opportunities and challenges came my way. When I was chairman of my hospital OB-GYN Department for four years there were many additional responsibilities, meetings and duties that came with the title. Our department had established a set of criteria regarding hospital charts and cases that required automatic peer review. If there was less than an adequate outcome in either an obstetrical or gynecologic surgery case as defined by these agreed upon criteria, the chart needed peer-review that became my responsibility. After reviewing the chart, if the care appeared to be substandard, the staff physician was notified and asked to be in attendance at the monthly hospital department meeting for a detailed discussion of the case and corrective action if the rest of the department concurred. The fact that these were colleagues that I saw regularly in the hospital and who elected me for the position didn't make the job any easier. Potential restriction of hospital privileges was always a touchy issue. My partners and I were subject to the same peer review by other staff members if one of our charts was reviewed for established criteria. These meetings were reminiscent of my days back at Pennsylvania Hospital where daily peer review by the Chief of Staff was a way of life. I was comfortable in this role. As a result, I suppose by reputation, over time medical malpractice defense attorneys began to hire me as an expert witness defending other OB GYN physicians who had a malpractice claim filed against them.

One such case was filed against a friend and neighbor of mine. He had done a suction D and C on a patient who miscarried. Because he was not an abortion provider, he had little experience doing this procedure on a pregnant uterus, much softer than a non-pregnant uterus. He inadvertently perforated the uterus with a suction cannula that then went into the patient's abdomen and suctioned the appendix off the intestine. He realized this immediately when he saw the appendix at the end of his suction cannula. Had he purposely tried to do this it would have been next to impossible to accomplish – just one of those bad outcome events that didn't necessarily imply medical malpractice. The patient needed emergency abdominal surgery. He did this surgery immediately with a general surgeon and months later the woman required a hysterectomy as well. The patient sued him and I was retained to help defend him as the medical expert. This was my first foray into the medical malpractice arena as an expert witness. We successfully defended him because although she had sustained injury, it was a recognized complication of the procedure and was handled appropriately and immediately without delay. On the one hand it was always important to show concern and compassion for the patient in front of the jury no matter what the injury. It was also important to balance this with the medical facts and recitation of what the Standard of Care required of the physician once the complication occurred. It was a fine line to walk in front of the jury from the witness stand while seated just feet in front of them. They watched every emotion from the expert in front of them, as well as listened intently to every bit of medical information explained to them in layman's terms so they could understand the case better. As the years went by, I became more involved and accomplished in the medical malpractice area. I found that I enjoyed the work and the drama of the courtroom, and that I was an effective expert witness for the defense. For me, it was a chance to show my professionalism, spontaneity, ability to communicate extemporaneously, challenge attorneys face to face who often thought they knew more medicine than I did, and a chance to help my peers. It was also a chance for my legal genes to express themselves.

The year after I stopped my clinical practice and before we moved from Arizona to Colorado I was retained by the Arizona Board of Medical Examiners to review obstetrical and gynecologic physicians who had come before the Board for potential discipline for one reason or another. At the Board's request I offered my opinions as to whether Standard of Care had been met in the case at hand before they decided on what if any restrictions to place on the physician's practice or license. I also had the opportunity to serve on a committee sponsored by the Mutual Insurance Company of Arizona and the Arizona Medical Association to review and advise on the merits of cases against their insured physicians.

When I later decided to hang out a consulting shingle on the Internet after retiring from active practice it didn't take malpractice plaintiff's attorneys long to find me. I was sent many cases to review, most of which I rejected because I saw no deviation from Standard of Care. Frankly, most of the Plaintiff's attorneys compensated me simply to find out their case had no merit. When a potential plaintiff came to them with a case, the attorneys, who were not medical experts by training or license, could not decide if the standard of care had been violated. That required an expert witness. But when told they had no case, as I often did when I reviewed the chart, they cut their financial losses and time and moved on.

Then there were those cases where upon my review Standard of Care had been violated and caused injury, and in my opinion those cases should move forward through the system as it existed. I, like most physicians, was not enamored with the medical malpractice system. The system had many faults and needed to be changed, but I was never in a position to change the system so I worked within its constraints. Frankly, if most hospitals had handled the substandard care within their own departmental committees as we did at the hospital where I was on staff, care would have been improved through local censorship and correction. But most physicians weren't interested in that kind of system or local pressure through peer review. There was too much turf protection going on. So cases wound up in the courts and expert witnesses were needed to move the cases forward. If the cases were not settled out of court then trial occurred in front of a jury. I had no trouble testifying against physicians who in my opinion fell below acceptable standards. It was really just an extension of Morning Report at Pennsylvania Hospital from years earlier, a necessary life long peer review process for me. Most of the cases that I did accept were settled outside of court, as they should have been, with the insurance companies paying on behalf of their insured physicians. But a few did go to trial in front of a judge and jury, and I did travel across the country for trials.

Some trials were more memorable than others. In one case in Colorado I told the lawyer he indeed had a good case from a medical standpoint, but if I were on the jury I wouldn't award more than $50,000 to the patient who had a surgical sponge left in her abdomen and required another surgery to have it removed. Sure there was an unnecessary surgery performed, and some additional loss of wages for a few weeks and some pain and suffering. Which is why if I were on the jury, $50,000 seemed reasonable to me. After expenses, it hardly seemed worthwhile to take the case in my humble opinion. He rightfully advised me that was not for me to decide. He obviously thought otherwise, took the case and a jury rendered a $1million verdict. My role had nothing to do with the jury deciding how much money to award.

That part of the trial was left to other actuarial and financial witnesses, and ultimately to the jury behind closed doors. Clearly the medical facts of the case were presented well to the jury. That was my role.

Compensation for the Plaintiff's attorney is usually through a contingency fee. This means no up front charges to the injured patient, but if a jury award comes back, the plaintiff's attorney receives an up-front agreed upon percentage of the award. The attorney was usually responsible to pay out of pocket expenses to get the case to trial, including expert witness hourly fees. But as one can see, if an attorney is getting 33% or more, they do quite well in a successful medical malpractice case. Their financial incentive is to take a case with merit, and to pursue it to a jury if necessary. On the other hand, the defense attorneys hired by the physician's malpractice carrier are paid by the hour, so they have no financial incentive to settle a case early in the process and will often not deal with a settlement offer until right before trial, often to maximize their own reimbursement through hourly charges. The trial lawyers tend to support the Democratic Party through political donations; thus the Democrats have little interest in changing the system as it is because of considerable trial lawyer lobbying money. Conversely, the Republicans support business, in this case the insurance industry, and lobby hard for change so that the insurance companies can be more profitable. Definitely this is a bad system all the way around, for everyone involved, and fraught with abuse. There needs to be a better solution. It is a crisis from every conceivable angle. As my Dad used to say all the time, ' If you don't like a law, change it. In the meantime, it is still the law."

Many have asked me why as a physician I even participated in this awful system. The system was going to continue whether or not I participated, and there were indeed physicians out there doing some rather unbelievable things to patients in a substandard fashion that was clearly wrong. Somehow they had to get the message to change their ways otherwise their substandard care would continue uncensored. I had no problems telling them that at deposition or trial, since they weren't hearing it from anyone else. Which is why many of the cases I accepted settled out of court, because during my deposition the physicians heard what I said under oath, and didn't want a jury to hear it. For those that were obstinate, a jury did hear it. That was within their control, but they chose to fight on.

In another case in upstate New York the elderly lawyer who retained me appeared to me to be slowing down mentally, but he had a good case if he could get the facts in front of the jury. Over the years I learned important questions that needed to be asked by the attorney to get relevant information to the jury. I told the plaintiff's attorney in no uncertain terms the questions he had to ask me, since there was no other way to get the important facts in front of the jury for them to hear unless he asked the questions. I couldn't volunteer the information in answer to un-related questions. That would trigger an objection from the defense attorneys. Clearly the other side wasn't going to ask the questions if the plaintiff's attorney didn't. He agreed to ask the questions. By the time we were given the only break while I was on the witness stand he still hadn't asked the relevant questions, so I reminded him during break one last time how important it was. When I went back on the witness stand he again didn't ask. He went blank. As a result this lawyer lost his own case. I knew it the minute I got off the witness stand. Some things were out of my control in the courtroom, for sure. There are many reasons why defense lawyers will take cases to the jury even when the facts are not on their side; knowing who their opponent is can be one of them. It is difficult to win a malpractice case against a physician. Juries are usually prone to side with the physician. There were times while I was being questioned by the defense attorney during trial in a case, even though there were no facts to support his side, the only defense for the physician was to make me look bad by attacking me as the expert. Of course, I had nothing to do with the patient's care and had only been retained as the expert witness.

Early in my malpractice expert witness career, in an effort to distract the jury from the facts of the case, one small town lawyer picked apart my resume discussing periods, commas, dates etc. that had been incorrectly typed, pointing out to the jury that I, too, made mistakes which I couldn't deny. He didn't ask me a single question about the case and won the case. I went back over my resume afterwards with a fine-toothed comb. It was unfair for the jury to decide this case against the plaintiff because a lawyer ridiculed me on the stand and didn't spend a moment on the medical facts of the case, but sometimes that is the way things worked out. Such was the nature of the beast. If the facts aren't on your side, attack the plaintiff's expert. At least the physician heard what I had to say from the witness stand. That in itself may have contributed to better medical care for his patients in the future. It wasn't always about who won or lost in front of the jury.

In one other case in Arizona, the defense lawyer told the jury that I said something in my earlier pre trial deposition that I knew for a fact I had not said since it was against my medical opinion and training. I was so outraged that without thinking and without knowing if I could even do what I was about to do, I swiveled in my chair from the witness stand and addressed the judge. I told him face to face that the attorney had just lied. There were a few moments of silence. Then the judge told the lawyer to go to my deposition, read the 10 lines before and 10 lines after the statement in question to the jury out loud. The lawyer was red faced, had lied as I said, and the case was over. No one believed any thing the lawyer said after that. This was courtroom drama, the kind of things juries loved – the unexpected.

I, too, had one case against me during my 25-year career that I authorized a payout from the insurance company on my behalf. A woman had come to me for an early first trimester pregnancy termination that was successfully completed by visual inspection and documented. She was given written instructions to follow before her return to see me in three weeks for a final checkup. Prior to that checkup she went to San Diego with her family and camped out. She felt ill. Her family left her alone and went to McDonald's to get her some food thinking it would settle her stomach. When they returned the woman was in cardiac arrest and undergoing care by the paramedics. She hemorrhaged into her abdomen from a ruptured tubal pregnancy.

She had both a combined intrauterine pregnancy that had indeed been terminated, and a concurrent tubal pregnancy that later ruptured. Due to hemorrhagic shock from blood loss, she suffered brain damage but lived because of good care she received at the hospital in California. The family sued me for missing the tubal pregnancy. In medical parlance she had what was called a combined heterotrophic pregnancy, which means a concurrent tubal and intrauterine pregnancy, a 1/40,000 occurrence. But it happened under my watch. My lawyer, one of the best defense lawyers in Phoenix at the time, gave me a 95% chance of winning the case in front of a jury and a 5 % chance of losing with the small risk of an award exceeding the $1million limits of my insurance policy. Given those good odds, I asked the insurance company to cover me in excess of my limits should that be necessary and we would go to trial and in all likelihood win. They refused. I authorized settlement. She and her family were awarded money from my malpractice carrier, perhaps as it was intended. I was initially distraught about the fact I felt backed into a corner and my insurance carrier would not accept my request. As time wore on I came to realize that this is why we as physicians have malpractice insurance. We needed peace of mind so that we could go on caring for patients on a daily basis and not have to worry about outcomes that we cannot predict and at times cannot prevent.

The other side of the coin was that female plaintiff's malpractice attorney's were women and needed obstetrical and gynecologic care like every other woman. Many OB GYN physicians just would not accept them as patients. Once I accepted one they seemed to flock my way. It was a small closely knit community that self-referred. After all, as women they required obstetrical care just like anyone else, as per my medical philosophy, so it was never an issue for me. One particularly notorious and successful plaintiff's attorney showed up on my doorstep to interview me to see if she wanted me to be her obstetrician. I must have passed the sniff test.

She was a control freak. I told her that when she was in my office she was not controlling the shots. I asked her what she did when she got on an airplane, whether or not she sat in the passenger seat or flew the plane? She understood the analogy. The attorney was over the age of 35, had a fibroid uterus, and she needed a genetic amniocentesis, which I performed in my practice. She was not married, and revealed nothing to me about the father of the baby. When she was lying on the exam table preparing for the ultrasound prior to the amniocentesis, I pulled down her panty hose with her permission and assistance to thigh level, sterilized the abdomen and draped her, drew up a local anesthetic into the syringe that I held above her thigh. As I unscrewed one needle from the syringe to replace it with another, I literally dropped the needle 90 degrees straight into her thigh where it took root. If I had taken aim at a bull's eye on the dartboard with a dart, I had a better chance of success than repeating what I had just done. There it was for all to see, no less with blood running down her thigh under her panty hose. Rather nonchalant, I said, "Look, if you are going to sue me just get it over with now." She laughed and we got on with it. Months later she came into the office in labor. I called over to Labor and Delivery to inform them that Nan was on her way over and in active labor. "Make sure Nan gets put into a room right away and on a fetal monitor," I said. I explained to the labor and delivery nurse with 25 years of experience that this patient was a malpractice attorney. The nurse said " We are busy, we have no rooms available right now, she will have to labor on a gurney in the hallway until a room is available, and I don't' give a shit who she is." It was just one of those days. She actually delivered on the gurney without complications. Against all hospital rules, I saw her later that night walking the halls with her Mom each sipping champagne from glass flutes. She was back in control, and I was happy all had ended well for her and her baby, and that she would forever be on my side.

One day when making hospital rounds, I sat at the nurse's station next to an elderly obstetrical colleague of mine who told me he had just been named in a malpractice suit. He was severely depressed as it was, his wife having recently died from ovarian cancer; this lawsuit did not help his mood any. What made this case interesting was that a gentleman who had just turned 20 years old, a man whom my colleague had delivered 20 years earlier, filed the lawsuit against him. Arizona, as happens in many states, has a law that says if a minor sustains a medical injury, he retains the right to file a law suit up to two years past the age of majority which means two years past the age of 18. Thus one week before his 20th birthday he filed this lawsuit against my colleague claiming injury to his arm resulting from a difficult shoulder dystocia injury at his birth 20 years earlier. It dawned on me that this, too, could someday happen to me. Which meant that if I stopped delivering babies when I was 50 years old, I would remain liable until I was age 70!

Chapter 10 Family Life

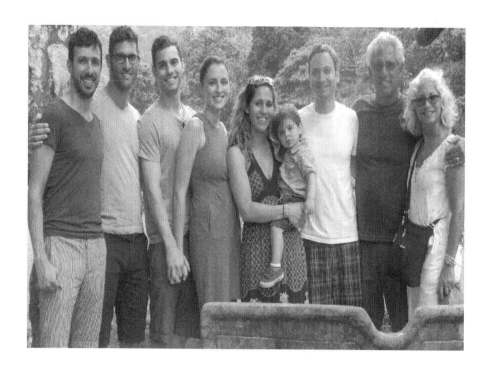

(El Valle, Panama, 2015)

During my last year of medical school I met my future wife who was then a student at the Hahnemann school of Allied Health. We met in front of a spiked punch bowl. I struck up the short-lived conversation that must not have been too impressive, because Julie doesn't remember the encounter. The next time we met was in a pub near medical school called Doc Watson's. I was having a few beers one night with classmates as she flew in and out. I made some comment to my friend about how 'hot' she was, and with the aid of a few beers under his belt he took the opportunity to blurt it out in public, to her embarrassment and mine. She does remember that encounter. Thank goodness for beer!

One evening a friend of hers called and told Julie to hurry to the medical school library where I was studying late one night. We had both been 'eyeing' each other at Hahnemann where she was a laboratory technician student before beginning her first career in special hematology and oncology research. In the library that night we connected after the hastily arranged meeting. Interestingly, we learned that we were both half Hungarian by birth and genetics, one of many things we would later discover we had in common. We were both of the same religion. We both wanted a family. We both were involved in health care professions and cared deeply for others above self.

Unfortunately I was juggling a few other women at the time, and it took longer than I would have liked to get back to her, which I did in due course. We dated most of my 4th year of medical school and fell in love, me first, she later. I can't say why she fell in love with me because I was difficult and focused on my career. But for me, aside from the obvious physical attraction, as we came to know each other better, I loved her sense of humor, her warmth, her effervescent personality, her smile, her scent, her drive and independence, her maternal instinct, and the way she carved a path for herself in life despite rather overwhelming family odds. Julie, on the other hand, needed more time where I was concerned. I was patient and waited for her, and gave her time and freedom to do as she pleased. We finally became engaged right before both of our graduations, she from the Allied School of Health Program at Hahnemann Medical College. We struggled to maintain some normalcy in our relationship during our one-year engagement while I interned at Pennsylvania Hospital and she worked with oncology physicians at Jefferson Hospital.

I would never encourage anyone to start a relationship during a year of medical internship. It was a brutal year, on call and up every third night all night for basically 36 hours straight, asleep immediately after and sometimes during dinner the next night, then one night off and awake before doing it all over again month after month for 12 months. She was a trooper putting up with my life, but such is the training for an OB-GYN physician and life to come. It took a special kind of woman to put up with the lifestyle. My feeling was if we could make it through internship year, we would make it through most anything else. 37 years later, three kids, one grandchild and another on the way, countless dogs (9 I think), living in four different States, career changes for both of us, subsequent bachelor and Master's degrees for her we are still thriving.

Julie is a very independent, strong willed, caring, gentle and loving person with an ebullient, effervescent personality. Stubborn, too, as am I, but we both think that can be a good thing and is from the Hungarian genes in us both. Her father was born in Budapest, Hungary and at the age of 13 wound up in Bergen-Belsen concentration camp for 4 years. He never much discussed those years with me, but one can only imagine the life long affect it had on him, which was obvious to us both in many ways. There has been much written about the children of Holocaust survivors, and indeed my wife was part of that community. Life with her father was not easy for her. Her mother was the daughter of Russian immigrants. Julie's parents lasted together for only a few years mostly because the only thing they had in common was dancing and music. Her childhood and upbringing were difficult and unstable, but to her credit, she made it work for herself from the time she was young. Thus her fierce independence and never say die attitude. I have always admired and loved her for her sense of independence, her undying spirit, her humor, her fortitude and perseverance, all of which were required to put up with me. Independence was necessary when married to a physician, especially one with a demanding career. We both wanted a family but put that off until my medical education was over. We correctly figured that it was best to spend a few years with each other before bringing kids into the world, knowing how our lives would change after children.

My wife and I had been trying to get pregnant
for over a year, unsuccessfully, during the fourth
and last year of my residency training. She only
ovulated a few times a year so timing was a bit
difficult, but we sure had fun trying. Fortunately
we only lived a block from the hospital, so when
ovulation happened, I ran back and forth. She
saw one of the infertility doctors on staff before
we left Philadelphia, and his advice was
prescient. "Forget about it for awhile," he said. "
Get set up out there in Phoenix, and if no luck see
someone then." So we forgot about it! I left my
long white coat, a symbol of the East coast
academia, behind. We were heading west. My
Chief of Service gave me a cowboy hat at a year-
end party! Off to Arizona we went, nomads that
we were to become, with not much other than
plants in our car and our heads full of medicine to
start a new life, hopefully a new family, and care
for women in Arizona. There was no way to
predict what was to come! But it was an exciting
time.

I had never driven across country. We had two weeks before I was expected at work, a new townhouse to set up, and a new city to learn. So we kept the medal to the pedal, as they say, which is the way I prefer driving anyhow. We took the southern route down the east coast, across the South, straight through Texas into New Mexico, then into Arizona. We drove about 8 hours each day, sometimes more. Texas was particularly difficult, never ending, and quite boring. As we headed in the westerly direction, the sun was constantly in our eyes and brutal. No surprise that as we look back on it, likely in Abilene, Texas where we stopped for some R and R, we conceived our first child. For a while after we had arrived in Phoenix we thought it was just the two of us until the nausea for Julie set in one day in the supermarket. Her periods were highly irregular anyhow, so it took us a while to figure it out. There was always more to learn about pregnancy no matter how much one thought he knew.

As expected, Phoenix in early July was hot. As the Phoenicians say, " But it is dry heat!" It kind of reminds me of opening a 400-degree oven door and being hit with a wall of dry heat in the face. Over time one does get used to it. For us, living there without access to a pool was unthinkable. Fortunately our townhouse complex had one. We were in the pool every day. We learned that all errands had to be completed quickly by 11 AM. We also learned to be careful when touching the car door and leather car seats. Air conditioning was an essential godsend to live in the desert.

So I assumed the position of attending Obstetrician and Gynecologist in private practice. I had a three-year contract leading to a buy-in as partner at the end of the third year if all went well. One of three physicians in this young practice, I immediately delved into the patient population affording my partners immediate time off to travel. Each went to Europe for three weeks, one right after the other, which essentially left me on call every other night for the first six weeks. But we all bonded well and I was happy.

Julie switched careers after a four-year stint in the oncology offices in Philadelphia. In addition to being a full time actively involved mother she went back to school and got a degree in Studio Art at Arizona State University, chipping away at it one course at a time, year by year. She had always had an interest not only in making art but also becoming an art therapist which she did later in life after getting a Master's Degree in Counseling and Art Therapy. Interestingly Hahnemann Medical College, where we met, had one of the first Art Therapy programs in the United States. Although interested when we were there, she learned that she didn't have the pre-requisites at the time.

My oldest son Jason was and still is a most interesting kid. From the onset of a difficult labor through birth by Cesarean requiring all of my skills to extract him, he was a challenge. As first time parents, we had no idea what to expect. He did not come out with a manual at the time of birth, and even though I was an Obstetrician, and a physician, and could take care of the sickest of sick babies at birth and in the NICU, it didn't mean that I knew anything about being a parent. We just assumed all babies were like him. We struggled to figure him out. Fortunately we are both mild mannered most of the time because he was impossible to figure out. I just remember being exhausted all the time. Night call was bad enough, but then throw in a kid who doesn't sleep and complained in one form or another about most anything, at all hours of the day and night, and well – it was a challenge. At 2 AM, when screaming for unknown reasons, the only thing that worked was to put him in his car seat and take him for a car ride. He fell asleep immediately but as soon as I pulled back into the garage, the screaming started all over again. We used to tell people we wanted four kids, and after him we narrowed it down to three. We loved him from the get go, and he was loads of fun, smart, challenging, inquisitive, and demanding. We gave him all of our attention, perhaps even too much of it, but who knew? He had so many varied interests and talents growing up that we had no idea where he would wind up or what he would do, but safe to say he is now a happy and content adult, with a great job making a difference in renewable energy and public policy, good friends, and no surprise, a fierce sense of independence for which we are more than half responsible. He is also a talented artist with his own studio producing wonderful works of art.

Our middle child Katie Rose is a girl. Everyone should have a daughter, but particularly an OB-GYN physician. There was always something to learn from every female in life. She was an absolute delight as a little baby, cute as a button, and sweet. She had me from the moment of birth. And everyone loved little Katie. She, too, was as independent as they come from the time she passed go, and put up with nothing from her older brother. Whatever he dished out, she gave right back. As a little girl of three or four I can still picture her walking around in our back yard in her cowboy boots with no clothes on. My Mom used to beg us to "Do something with her hair" because she never let anyone touch it, so it was always wild. Finally, one day I just told my Mom that if it bothered her, she could do what she wanted with Katie's hair. She learned! Somewhere around this time we got a call from the day care center telling us they wanted to talk to us about her. They were concerned because she was telling all the kids in her class how the egg and sperm met and that was where babies came from. I asked them if they knew whether she got it right. I was proud of her then as I am now. They thought we needed to talk to her and I explained I already had which was why she was educating the rest of her preschool class. She clearly has figured out now, as she had then, how to give us grandchildren!

Katie loved the back yard swimming pool and took to it like a fish. The drain in the deep end of the pool was at 10 feet depth. She used to put her little arms around my neck, and we would go down there and just sit with my fingers placed in the drain to hold on until I couldn't breath any longer, then we would come back up together. She had an amazing set of lungs that she would use to belt out a scream that could shatter a glass. We also used to take her to a community pool with a high dive. People thought we were nuts to let her climb up by herself, which she did as a little 4 year old, then stand at the end of the diving board all by herself. When she was ready, she jumped.

Later in life I had occasion when she was in middle school to talk to her class about what it was that I did in life. I began by asking someone to come up to the board and try to write 'Obstetrician and Gynecologist' on the blackboard. Seeing no volunteers, I of course picked on her. She almost got it right, spelling

'Gynacologist' incorrectly. She still has not forgiven me for correcting her in front of her classmates. After the session was over she informed me all the boys in the class came up to her and told her how cool it was that I got to look at naked women all day long. I don't think she was too happy about that either. In their minds, that is what I did. Boys will be boys! I didn't have the heart to tell them that not everyone looked so good naked. That was for them to find out some day. She also has a great story about her first pelvic exam, but we need not go into that one.

Our daughter loved the theater arts, so no surprise that she majored in this field in college, then headed to LA for fame, fortune, hard work, and waitressing. While I considered the operating room my theater, I would never be caught on a real stage with real lights shining on me as she did. Stage fright personified would be how best to describe it for me. Although one on one, I do at times have a sense of the dramatic in me, as she quickly points out to me at times: "And you wonder where I got it from" is how she puts it. She played the piano and sang a beautiful love song to her husband on their wedding day in front of the crowd. Today she is an actress with a steady salaried full time position in theater doing what she loves. For us, we couldn't be more proud of her for pursuing her dreams, and for producing a great grandson for us, the first of more, we hope.

We took a respite for a while from the baby making business to get a handle on our changing and expanding lives. We moved into a larger home after a few years in a residential neighborhood with good primary schools, and decided to keep our kids in the public school system, a decision we never regretted. Our sense of it was that if they were smart, capable students, they would shine no matter where they were, which proved to be true. The kids participated in all kinds of after school and weekend activities which we attended regularly.

T Ball, boys' baseball and girl's softball games, swim meets, gymnastics and ice skating lessons, piano recitals, tennis, children's theater performances, lacrosse, etc.

In the early days before cell phones I carried a beeper that meant that it just went off, with no text message. So I would have to drive to a pay phone, call the answering service, then call the patient or the hospital, and return to the event whenever possible, only to go through the whole process all over again, sometimes minutes later. One can understand then how excited I was when the first Motorola cell phone came out, for which I paid $2000. I would have paid more just so I could sit and watch a baseball game at the field in peace.

As it is with all children, so too was our youngest son Zachary a gift, or as he calls himself a "walk in the park", compared to his older siblings. By now we were experienced and at

ease with parenting, and perhaps that had
something to do with his personality. But I just
think he was a sweet kid from day one. He was
also very observant, and learned quickly what
would get him in trouble just by watching his
older siblings, both of whom adored him. He
enjoyed life, his home life, his siblings, his dogs,
and his friends. He had boundless energy that
often bounced off the walls, resulting in calls
from school, most of which got overlooked by his
teachers because he was cute. As for his friends
who were most important to him, here are their
comments about his Dad "I was always very
proud of the fact that my dad was a doctor, but
when I explained to my friends what he did, it
was often greeted with the predictable 'Eww,
your dad looks at vagina's all day?'" As
hormones started to change a bit, their
responses inevitably migrated to: 'Cooool, your
dad looks at vagina's all day!' Fortunately for me,
I usually held the ultimate trump card against
potential bullying since it was often their mom's
vaginas I was looking at in my office.

As to what home life was like after a long day of work, his memories include: "After a long day at the hospital, he often came home and jumped in to the kitchen, sometimes still in his scrubs, to help mom with dinner and dishes before retiring to the couch. There, he would soon pass out from exhaustion while Jason, Katie and I took advantage of the situation and tortuously tickled his feet or plugged his nose to stop the snoring." Kids!

We certainly disrupted his emotional life in the summer between 8th and 9th grade, when we decided to sell our home in Phoenix after I retired and move away from all that he knew to the small mountain community of Telluride. He was angry at us, and depressed for most of his first year in high school, although we knew it was a good move for him because not only was it a better high school, but also he would get individual attention in small classrooms, more so than had he stayed at his large high school in Central Phoenix. There were definite advantages for our son, however, in being the new guy on the block in a small class that had pretty much known each other since grade school. It didn't take long for girls to find him, or for him to make life friends. He missed his lacrosse terribly, so his Mom took it upon herself to start what has turned out to be a very successful youth lacrosse program at Telluride high school that has long outlasted us there, a program that initially faced long odds of succeeding yet is thriving today. But my wife persisted because she knew how important it was for him. He learned how to ice skate, not a huge sport in Phoenix as one might imagine, but eventually he skated well for the local high school ice hockey team. He found his way onto the stage at the local opera house performing in school plays. In one he even dressed as a woman and belted out songs to the community. When he graduated, he took some pride in being able to say he made it through high school without ever finishing a book cover to cover, which although perhaps true, certainly didn't hold him back. He pursued a successful undergraduate degree in Advertising in the Big Ten, has been gainfully employed in Chicago ever since, and is now well on his way to getting an MBA at night school while working during the day. In the end, the move was a good one for him, as even he will now admit.

I asked him for his thoughts about what it was like for him to grow up the son of an OB GYN physician. He got to know me from a unique perspective, both at the end of my career and at the beginning of the next phase of my life. "My dad has always said the reason he went in to Obstetrics was because it is one of the few medical practices that dealt primarily with happy occasions. For the most part, childbirth is a joyous time for women and the overwhelming expectation is that all will go well and a healthy child will be welcomed in to the world. However, when things go wrong, the delicate balance of life can be immediately shifted from elation to tragedy. That fear must be a high motivator for all obstetricians, and, for my dad, I believe it metastasized to a pursuit of perfection and intense attention to detail; qualities that span far beyond his work. He dedicated countless hours to preparing for all scenarios in a profession that leaves little margin for error; it must have been nearly impossible to turn off that part of his brain. Unless we had escaped to the mountains of Telluride, when my dad was practicing, he was never really able to build a clear buffer between his occupation and the rest of his life. For better or worse, being an OBGYN doc defined him. No one will ever accuse my dad of being overly in-tune with his feelings, and I would deduce that the decades protecting himself from the nastier side of medicine greatly contribute to that. Because there was always potential for tragedy and heartbreak in the medical profession, I imagine many docs perfect the ability to remove emotion from harsh situations. I'm sure my dad put up a huge emotional shield at work; if he hadn't, there likely would have been great potential for the dark-side of obstetrics to completely decimate his mental well-being. With that said, I'm sure many doctors deal with similar situations in far more destructive ways. Fortunately, there are many redeeming qualities he needed in the OR that translated positively to parenting. Confidence, composure and the ability to clearly articulate any situation likely came in handy when dealing with three wily children."

He was right. Compartmentalizing emotions and feelings was a necessary evil of being a physician. Although I rarely showed it, I felt emotions every waking hour of every day. It was impossible not to when exposed to raw emotions from patients every day. There was a fine line to walk, honed after years of experience, between being empathetic and able to help patients through their given situation in life, and coming home daily an emotional, exhausted wreck. I had my own family and life to be a part of, and I needed to keep myself in a zone where I could be a committed, loving parent and husband, and put the emotional trauma of the day somewhere else. For my wife, a very emotional being, it required a lifelong effort to help me get in touch with my emotions; an effort that is ongoing to this day. I am still working at it!

From the time before our first son was born, my wife and I were dog people. We eventually wound up with the miniature Schnauzer breed. When my family was spending the summer in Telluride Colorado and I was commuting back and forth to Phoenix, I took the occasion to see some newborn Schnauzer puppies. But which one to choose?   I sat in the back yard of the breeder's house and just watched them play. The first one that came up to me, crawled up on my lap and licked my nose was the eventual winner. Rosie, as she came to be called, chose me first.

Several years later, when my children were young teenagers, we decided to mate Rosie with another purebred miniature Schnauzer, Sonny.

Sonny and his handler came over to our backyard on the appointed day as we all sat around the kitchen table to watch the big event. For most of the first hour they danced around each other with no contact, until finally the handler went out and told Sonny to get to work. He listened. My kids called it rape, but it did result in a successful pregnancy for Rosie. It also gave us the opportunity to talk about sex, sexually transmitted diseases, and contraception. After all, why not take advantage of the opportunity! Several weeks later I took a pregnant Rosie into my office, laid her on her back for about ten seconds while I performed a quick ultrasound. It looked like we were going to have a litter of six.

We spent weeks preparing a delivery room for her in a small bathroom next to our bedroom where she slept in her dog bed. I had string to tie the umbilical cords, hemostats to prevent bleeding after the cords were cut, towels, scissors, and anything else I could think of. I had never assisted a dog in labor or birth, but I felt appropriately credentialed to carry it off. One early morning my wife and I were awakened early to a strange noise. We jumped out of bed to go see what Rosie was up to. When we opened the bathroom door, there she was sitting in her doggie bed surrounded by six nursing puppies. There was not a drop of blood or placenta to be found anywhere. She had a look of exhaustion, satisfaction and pride on her face. I was dumbfounded. How was it that a dog could do this on her own, deliver sextuplets, with an obstetrician in the next room, not awaken me or ask for help? What was it that I had been doing incorrectly all these years? The puppies were the cutest and we loved them to death for the next two months. We kept one, Lucy, who went on to live with us for the next 15 years.

I delivered so many babies in a rapidly growing Phoenix, Arizona that I developed a strong desire for anonymity and privacy. It was hard to go anywhere without a big 'hello' from someone and a "do you remember when you delivered…"

which I rarely did. It was always difficult for me to go to the Price Club because it seemed everyone who worked there or shopped there was a patient. So I began to seek out Nature more and take family trips and vacations to remote out of the way places where I could go unrecognized. Once when skiing in Show Low, Arizona on the Apache reservation, we stopped to fill the car with gas in one of the most out of the way places anyone could ever be. As the tank was filling I draped myself over the hood of the car and caught a few rays of sun before the long drive home. 'Hi Doc!!" came a loud shout of recognition and a big wave from someone driving by on the highway. I was found once again!

I was known as one of the few physicians in Arizona who didn't golf. Frankly, I didn't have the time and preferred any down time with my family. I was constantly driving back and forth to the hospital for deliveries, day and night, although it was only a short five-minute drive. Vacation time was always a welcome respite.

Because we had a group practice and covered for each other when we were gone it was relatively easy to get away and leave the office behind. After my wife and I had seen the Grand Canyon for the first time we both agreed that the only way to really appreciate it was from the Colorado River way down in the depths of the Canyon.

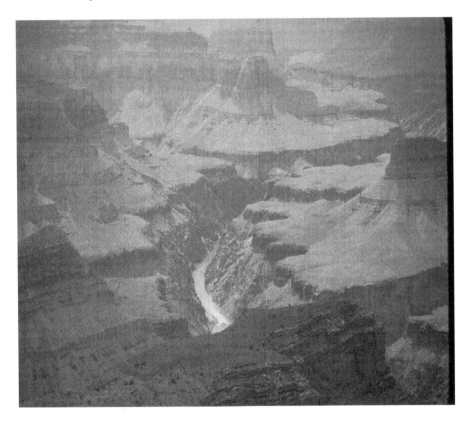

We signed up way in advance for a River Rafting

trip since there was a wait and only so many people per year were allowed on the River. When we got the call we had two kids at the time. My parents had since retired to Arizona (they found out where Arizona was and loved it). We left the two little ones with them for eight days and disappeared into the depths of the Canyon with no way of communication to or from the outside world. My parents never forgave us for that, accusing us of abandoning our children. "And what would you do if something happened to them while you were down there?" my mother queried. I told her we would find out about it when we came back. Besides, it was much more likely something would happen to us than to them. She wasn't reassured. But there are just some things you only get to do once in life!

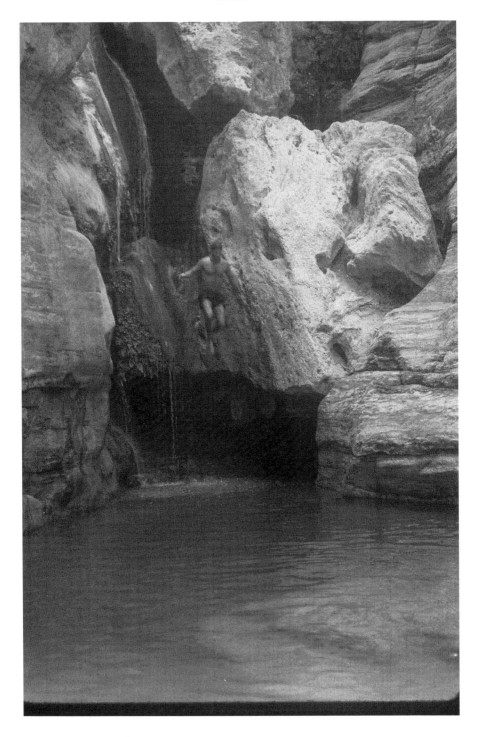

So off we went, boarding our raft at the base of the Glen Canyon dam and Lake Powell, exiting at Temple bar and flying a little puddle jumper into Las Vegas over Lake Meade. We saw the whole Canyon form one end to the other, over 300 miles. What a glorious wonder it was!

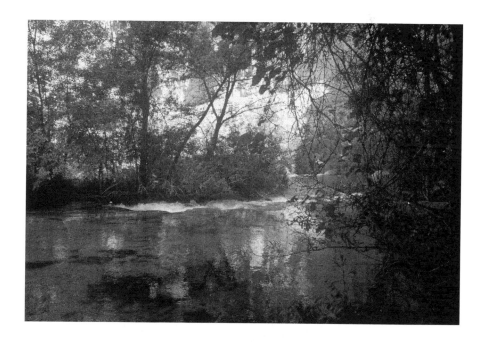

The Colorado River was ice cold as it shot out from the bottom of the Glen Canyon dam and

Lake Powell. Fortunately for us it was early summer. We took quick baths in the River that took our breath away, welcome respite from the heat that it was.

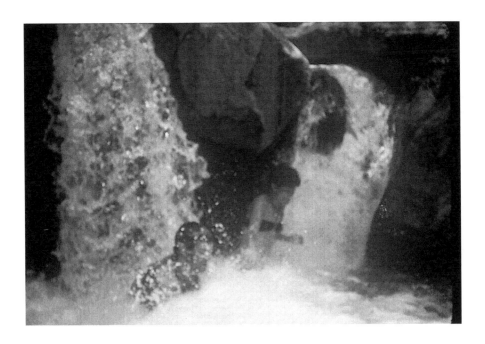

We went over Lava Falls and Crystal rapids, considered the big ones. I rode the pontoons of the raft the whole time and at one point wound up in the frigid rapidly flowing river before I was extracted and placed back in the raft. There was a whole group of young and virile New York fireman on the rafts with us, as well as a mixed group of all kinds of people from everywhere. Havasupai canyon was extraordinarily beautiful.

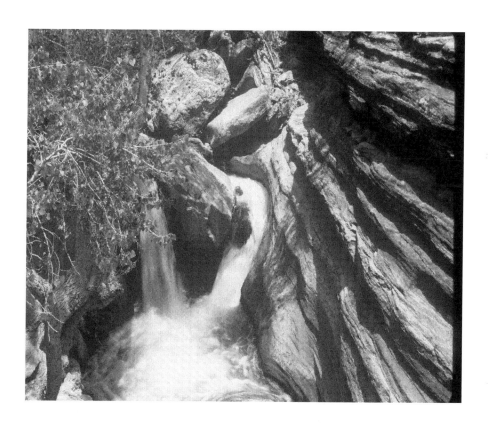

Waterfalls were abundant and gorgeous.

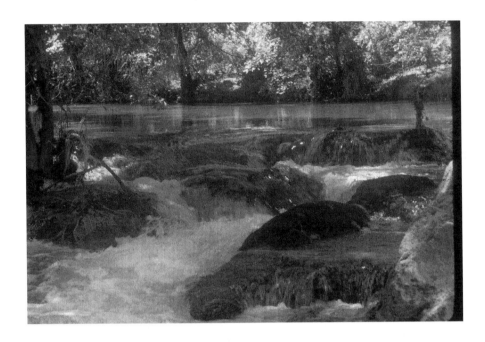

Day hikes up to some narrow trails on the cliffs were spectacular if not dangerous. Camping out on the small beaches at night in tents next to sheer cliffs of granite would occasionally lead to the death of some unfortunate people every year.

This trip was a memorable birthday for me. The fright began when we were camping one day after a full day of rafting. While we were on the little sandy beach Julie disappeared. I couldn't find her anywhere and there were only a few places to look. Nightfall was setting in early as it did in the bottom of the narrow canyon. I paced the small beach from one end to the other, several times, and she was nowhere to be found. I peered into as many tents as I could. I thought maybe she hooked up with one of the fireman. I just didn't know what else to think other than the river took her away when suddenly she appeared from behind some big rocks at the end of the beach where she went for a few moments of privacy, skinny-dipping, and meditation. I was not happy! But I was overjoyed that she was alive. So it made it difficult to appreciate the Dutch oven birthday cake the river rats made for me that evening.

The trip ended in Vegas where we took our first prolonged bath and shower in over a week. We had never been to Vegas before so it was new to us. A good nap, shower and down to the Hotel casino show. The noise, lights, loud music, bare-breasted women with tassels on their nipples, smoke, and general mayhem was so far removed from where we had been in the tranquility of Mother Nature with no lights, noise or electricity that it was true culture shock. We hopped the next plane out and got back to our life, children, dogs, and Phoenix.

My 40th birthday was also memorable. Julie had arranged to surprise me with a sailboat vacation in the Virgin Islands, the two of us on a boat with a captain and first mate. I had always wanted to spend time sailing. It was a wonderful thing she did by arranging this for us. For me, however, I had a problem with the passing of decades. And 40 seemed like it was the halfway point in life for me, so I had problems from the start with this birthday, not the trip. But off we went. It was a lovely time and a lovely 40-foot sailboat. The first night we anchored off a portion of Saint John Island in the evening. I didn't get a good look at the island until I awakened early in the morning. I went on deck around 6 am in my skimpy bathing suit, saw a beautiful isolated beach adjacent to the woods, dived off the boat and swam for five minutes to get there. When I arrived at the beach I laid back and enjoyed the pristine beauty, the birds chirping sweetly, the sailboat in the distance, and the privacy. Then I heard a voice with a deep-pitched English accent from somewhere in the woods behind me, " Get your bare white ass out of here". I struggled to see who it was. Through the trees I could see an old lady with a shotgun pointed right at me. Back in the ocean I went and swam back to the sailboat. Greetings from the Virgin Islands! A few days later on my actual birthday, we wound up in Virgin Gorda at a beautiful ocean resort and bar appropriately named the Bitter End Yacht Club. With gorgeous rock formations in the foreground and endless miles of sea green Ocean between Europe and us at this point, one could imagine being almost anywhere in the world but always at sea with countless more places to visit. I got loaded, just me and the other derelicts at the Bitter End Yacht club Bar! Welcome to the 40's! Julie says I never enjoyed the birthday trip, and she would never plan a birthday party for me again. I was glad about that but she was wrong about not enjoying the trip. It was great!

My quest for exploring Mother Nature, privacy, anonymity, and my love of skiing took me and my family all around the mountain West on snow skis – Aspen, Vail, Durango, A Basin, Crested Butte, Keystone, Park City, Taos, Jackson Hole, Buttermilk, Aspen Highlands, Steamboat, Flagstaff, and Telluride. My kids became expert skiers at a very young age. I kept in touch with Mother Nature this way and got myself recharged for going back to work. But increasingly I needed more time off. The day to day of long hours, a large patient load, long nights always on the alert and ready for action 24/7, managing partners and their idiosyncratic behavior, listening to petty staff issues daily, dealing with insurance or lack thereof, paying invoices and meeting payroll, rising malpractice insurance costs, and running a women's research business on the side was taking a toll on me although I was oblivious to it. Julie wasn't.

Telluride, Colorado had special appeal for all of us. The distance gave me respite from the phone calls. An eight-hour car drive from Phoenix through the Painted Desert and large Navajo reservation, just the drive alone was like finding Mother Nature all over again. It was as many before and after us called it, 'God's country'. I never minded the drive and did it countless times with kids, their friends, and dogs. It was also good bonding time with the family. We sang songs, played word games, laughed, ate beef jerky, and played with the dogs. "On the road again" by Willy Nelson became my theme song. "Just can't wait to get on the road again."

Located in the Southwestern corner of
Colorado near Four Corners area, surrounded by
14,000-foot peaks and some of the best skiing in
Colorado if not the world, Telluride was a small
mountain town in a box canyon. I considered it
the prettiest part of Colorado. Thus for me at
least it was the prettiest part of the country. It
was an extremely progressive and liberal
community much to my liking.

Arizona politics was increasingly bothersome
to me, too. Evan Mecham was an
archconservative millionaire car dealer and
inflammatory racist who was elected governor by
a 40% vote in a three-way race, then later
impeached. He called black kids 'pickaninnies'
and said Jews needed to face up to the fact the
US was a Christian nation. He said MLK was not
deserving of a holiday and ended it in Arizona.
Following him, J. Fife Symington, another
Republican and East Cost aristocrat, was elected

twice before a felony conviction for tax fraud. He, too, was removed from office. The Savings and loan debacle with Charlie Keating at the helm was nothing other than pure greed at its worst. Then there was and remains Sheriff Joe Arpaio and his prisoner tent colonies in the desert. I never really blamed the politicians. They were who they were. It was the people who kept electing them over and over again that I just couldn't fathom. That is what bothered me. Colorado increasingly looked more and more attractive to me.

It is said by locals that most people find Telluride in the winter because they ski there. Snow is abundant.

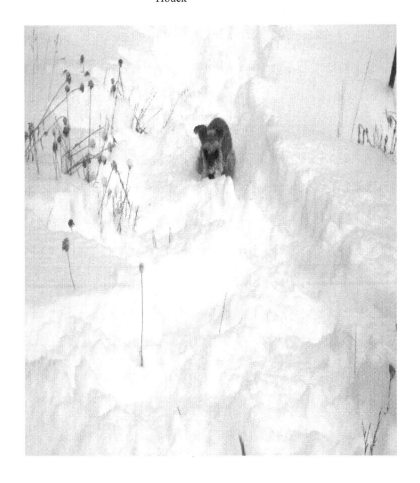

However, those who ultimately choose to live there find it because of the summer. One summer my wife and I did visit and really fell in love, so much so that we bought land at 10,000 feet above sea level in a beautiful aspen forest with a year long bubbling glacial creek adjacent to a ski run. For us it was initially just a land investment, but a magical one at that. We had no intention of ever living there or building a home there. But things have a way of changing.

One day around the age of 50 I came home to my wife who said: " Change your life, or change your wife." We had always been friends and still were. My health and our relationship were uppermost in her mind. She correctly sensed I was unhappy. I had gained weight. She said I looked gray and had one foot in the grave. I was in the prime of my medical career, at the top of my game, and felt like I still had much to offer my patients. It was me that I hadn't given much thought to over the years. It was always about someone else first. I had successfully learned how to compartmentalize my emotions, perhaps appropriate to practice good objective medicine, but not conducive to a good lasting personal relationship. I wasn't aware of my own feelings and dissatisfactions. As difficult as it was for me to do, after considerable thought and the realization that she was indeed correct, I decided

to walk away from it all. So I changed my life!
And she saved my life for the first time.

In the intervening years we had built a home
that we used as a vacation home on our property
in Telluride, Colorado. Now we decided to move
from Phoenix. We sold our home there, took a
year to unwind our professional and business
affairs, said good by to our friends who thought
we were insane to move to an isolated little ski
town in the mountains of Colorado, got in our car
with our kids and dogs, and off we went on
another nomadic journey. We said goodbye to
Arizona after 21 years in the desert.

Many of my patients were upset since I was
the only physician for whom they had 'assumed
the position', not an easy thing for any woman
with which to get comfortable. Most patients just
couldn't understand it and were not happy that
they would have to start over again with
someone else. I received many thoughtful and

loving cards when I left practice. There was one patient, though, who understood it quite well. She had been a patient of mine for years. Her father was in his early 70's and still practicing solo as a family physician in Phoenix. I always had the utmost respect for those physicians who could continue to practice solo and do so for that many years. It takes a very special, dedicated, and committed individual. She asked me how many years I had been practicing OB-GYN. I sat there on the exam room stool, thought about it, and replied 25 years. She looked me straight in the eyes and said, " That is a wonderful career, a long time, and you have every right to move on and do something else." As the daughter of a father who had not done so, she spoke from the heart and could empathize with me. I felt as if she had given me permission, that it was acceptable, and I should not be so hard on myself.

One of the many things that I learned as an obstetrician was the ability to see with clarity into the future, or at least 9 months into the future, and then make it come true. It is not something the average human being can do. All of my training, years of clinical experience and expertise was geared to producing a healthy baby and mother 9 months after they first appeared in my office as a unit. We look at numbers, examine patients, feel abdomens, perform ultrasounds, look at labs, listen to and measure babies one way or the other, all with the idea that everything must turn out perfectly 9 months down the road on separation from each other. There was no room for error. We think like this dozens of times a day, day in and day out, and do get to the point where the future is clear. This time, however, I had no idea what was to come next, which was both the fear and the excitement!

Chapter 11   Life after Private Practice

As a physician, there is really no such thing as life after medicine; once a physician, always a physician. The very word physician implies teaching, learning, sharing, healing. So it is not something one really ever walks away from when one decides to stop clinical practice. It becomes part of one's personality. It is rather a decision of how one chooses to live life now that circumstances have changed. What I knew was that I no longer wanted employees lives to manage any more; if I were to do anything I wanted to be solo. I no longer wanted a rigid schedule to adhere to. I no longer wanted to be indoors in an office all day, nor did I want to get into the elevator of my office building any more. I no longer wanted to be driving back and forth to the hospital night and day. I no longer wanted business partners anymore, other than my own family. But what did I want to do with my life? That took some thought. Spending time in Africa helped me sort out what I didn't want. I came to the realization that I still had an active license to practice medicine, I had a lot of medical information in my head, and I was still a physician. Truly, a medical degree and license are valuable documents to possess.

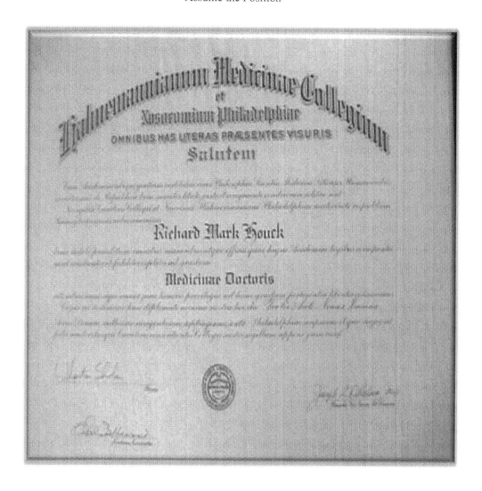

I was now living in Colorado, a great place for people with rugged individualism and independent spirit. Telluride, Colorado was one of the most politically liberal, progressive, beautiful communities in the whole State.

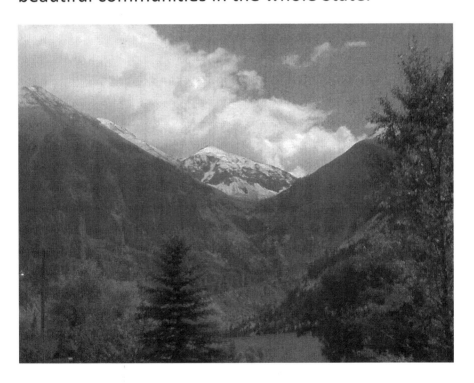

(Telluride, Colorado in the early fall.)

This is what appealed to me and was one of many reasons I continued to return there as I did from Africa for the next phase of my life. While I was gone my wife and youngest son, still at home, settled in for our new life. I reasoned that with all the famous names living full or part time in this small town, Dan Quayle, Norman Schwarzkopf, Tom Cruise, Laura Linney, Dick Ebersol, Oprah Winfrey, Richard Holbrooke, Clive Cussler, Meg Whitman, Oliver Stone, Sylvester Stallone, Ralph Lauren, Jerry Seinfeld, and those who visited like Andre Agassi, Steffi Graf, Lionel Ritchie, Donald Trump, Dennis Rodman, all of them but one for their own reasons wanted some peace and privacy in their lives.

The rest of the town folk respected the privacy of those they passed on the street, which was unique about this beautiful and isolated ski town. In town there were Swedes and Finns who resided here for generations, all from mining families. There were people who just loved living here because of the natural beauty of the place. There were hard-core naturalists and environmentalists, massage therapists, physical therapists, and alternative therapists. There were hippies and lots of fit young and old people alike who just wanted to ski, paraglide, hike, mountain climb and ice climb, to fly fish, snowmobile or ride horses. There were lawyers, doctors, investors, arms manufacturers, restaurateurs, realtors, bankers, cooks, waiters and waitresses, authors, politicians, and businessmen and women that were all essential to make a viable small town of 2500 people a mountain community with a great Main street that was very fun and functional. There was an exceptional high school and teachers. Telluride was often featured in commercials and movies simply because of its beauty. In the gorgeous mountain summertime there were lively festivals every weekend, from Mountain Film, to Bluegrass, Jazz, Chamber Music, Mushroom, Balloon, Wine, and the Telluride Film festival that annually brought the glitterati from Hollywood, New York and around the world to this mountain playground.

The one person who never seemed to fit was Stallone, who in the early days of Mountain Village bought up a huge number of lots for his friends and cronies. One large lot was reserved for his personal use and for his polo ponies. At the time when he bought all these parcels they were located on or around Tooth Street high in the Mountain Village, so named by the developer, a former dentist. Ski runs, Aspen trees, and large Colorado blue spruce trees surrounded the area adjacent to where my wife and I bought a parcel just before him.

It was never easy to say we lived on Tooth Street, anyhow. So we were happy with the new street name – Rocky Road. Not long after, Stallone picked up and left Telluride to move on to Aspen, more to his liking with more 'party' action and attention.

Telluride had a reputation for hosting one of the best 4th of July parades in the country. Excitement would mount in front of the courthouse on Main Street at 10:45 AM. During the time I lived there, General Norman Schwarzkopf would shake hands with the local Veterans who led the parade and the Pledge of Allegiance. The roar of two fighter jets would buzz the town at rooftop level and head straight to the end of the box canyon towards Ajax peak, a 14er, then shoot straight up at a 90 angle. It was a pretty awesome sight. I was always curious how this start for the 4th of July parade got arranged, who authorized it, and who other than us tax payers paid for the fuel. Yet it still was an awesome sight. Then the parade began. The main street was lined with chairs filled with families 7-8 deep from all over the state and surrounding states. Dogs and little kids on bikes decorated with red, white and blue streamers, floats with local bands and drums beating out a rhythm, Men without Rhythm dancing helter skelter in tune to no one (often local politicians), fire engines blaring their horns, town notables in open air classic vehicles, women of the Wild West dressed in 19th Century fashion riding side saddle on horses, Rowdy Roudebusch (a local cowboy), occasionally inebriated riding his stallion down the street and later into the Sheridan Bar for a drink – one after another, each a more colorful entry than the one before, the parade wound slowly down the Main Street. It was a hoot. When the parade was all over everyone headed to town-park for an old fashioned barbecue sponsored by the local volunteer fire department members who had earlier prepared and cooked the food. They raised money by donations for the evening's fireworks, a splendid array against the massive mountains, lit by stars and the moon. This was Telluride in all its summer glory.

The winter was simple; just snow, and lots of it, with great steep skiing right down into the town on the most infamous steep double black diamond ski run, the Plunge. For me, Milk Run and Bushwhacker were my favorite ski runs. There was a free gondola connecting the Town of Mountain Village to the Town of Telluride, one of the most awesome free rides anywhere in the Country. All in all, it was a special place with special people lucky enough to live there and they all knew it.

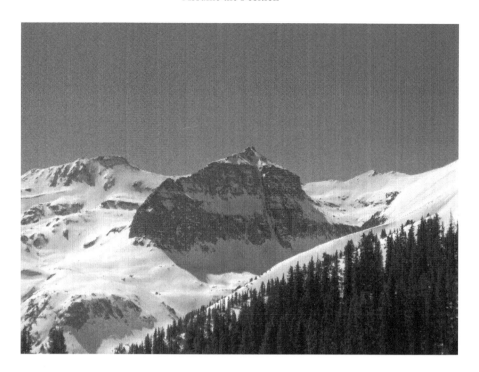

My wife and I were quick to meet people and make friends.

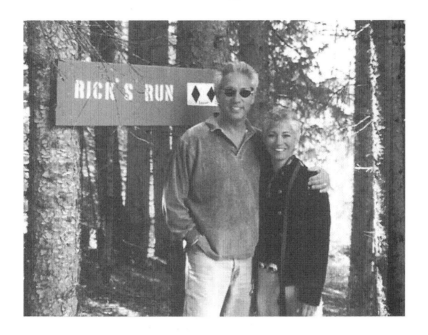

We volunteered for many local charities and
shared the philosophy that it was important to
leave a place even better than we found it. We
joined the Telluride Foundation, a non-profit that
raised funds for other non-profits and
organizations in the County. As a benefit we had
many occasions to ski what was referred to as
'First Tracks" before the mountain opened to the
general public, usually from 7-9 AM when no one

else was on the mountain. While the sun was just rising over the glorious mountain peaks, and the clouds were a beautiful pastel pink, it was often cold, frosty, but always pristine on the mountain at that time of the morning in midwinter. Then we would adjourn to someone's beautiful slope side home for breakfast and ski home by 11.

On one of these occasions we sat by a hot fire drinking hot chocolate. The presentation featured Franz Klammer, Olympic gold medalist, and Franz Weber, World speed skiing champion. Films of their great runs and brutal crashes were shown to pump everyone up before we left for the First Tracks skiing. As luck would have it I got on the same chair lift with one other fellow and the two Franz's. After brief introductions, I turned to Klammer, my skiing idol, and asked. "I have always wondered what goes through your head when you are skiing on the edge at 60-70 miles or more per hour, then you look down and realize there is only one ski on the ground, the other is out of control, and there is that split second before you realize you are going to crash?" He looked at Weber, then at me, and said one word – "Shit". We all laughed. For me, that resonated!

In my mind's eye, I pictured myself skiing like Klammer, though there was absolutely no comparison other than it was the way I wanted to ski and we each had a pair of skis on our feet. It was all about going straight down hill for me as fast as I safely could without falling or hitting a tree. As a friend of mine said about my skiing, " You were absent from ski class the day they talked about turning!" Fortunately I had good balance, because my form was severely lacking. But I was always smiling when on skis, the cold fresh mountain air on my face and in my lungs. It was exhilarating!

Most of my life, I felt much better being in

control. It didn't matter whether it was of my own emotions, choosing college courses that I knew were best for me and my chosen career, skiing my own way in my own style, or managing my patient's pregnancies and surgeries. I looked for ways that I knew would give the best outcome. I didn't mind being on the edge, or even not knowing what was coming next, because I trusted in my ability to keep things from getting out of control. I didn't like chaos and I didn't enjoy not having control of my life.

One early summer day while poking around outside our mountain home wearing my old smooth soled boat shoes from years earlier in the Virgin Islands, I decided at that moment I had to go up on the roof. It wasn't unusual for me to be on the roof of my home. I tinkered, cleaned gutters, cleaned sky light windows, fixed loose shake wood roof tiles, in the winter broke up ice dams and snow raked the roof. In general, my philosophy was that if I could do it myself there was no reason to pay someone else to do it. I enjoyed caring for our property and being outdoors anyhow, rain, snow, sunshine or sleet. I extended the ladder, placed it squarely against the back roof, and up I went. The roof itself, at its lowest point, wasn't that high above the ground from the back, maybe 10 feet or so, but from there up to the top of the vaulted ceiling where the sky lights were was a pretty good shot up. I remember poking around the skylight, and I remember looking down at my boat shoes. They were probably slipping at that point. The next thing I remember is being inside the CT scanner at the Telluride Medical Center. I remember bits and pieces of the ambulance ride to St Mary's hospital in Grand Junction, two and a half hours away. I vaguely remember yelling at some doctor whom I didn't know as she removed me from the operating table without performing the surgery that my wife had authorized. Clearly I was not in control, and I later was told that I was not nice about it.

My youngest son was in the kitchen watching

television and eating breakfast at the time I flew by the dining room window, head first aiming for the ground. He will tell you that I would do anything to avoid having him beat me in racquetball, which he has done once in his lifetime. We had a match scheduled for later that day. He was predictably quite distressed to see me plunge head first down in front of the kitchen window and was first on the scene to find me slumped on my back, unconscious and moaning. He immediately called 911. My wife trailed the ambulance up to our house, wondering the whole time where it was going. She was rather distressed to find it drove into our driveway. The paramedics apparently reassured my wife and son that I would live. As for me, I was clearly in neurogenic shock with a concussion, unconscious for most of the next several hours, and heavily sedated with narcotics. My memory of the whole event was clouded so that when I retell the story, I don't have the same fear as those who saw me. I don't think it was pretty, though, and left a traumatic visual image for my son as I plunged downward headfirst. My right wrist was shattered, my ribs were broken, and my right hip was fractured at the acetabulum. Obviously I was concussed. The good news was my neck was not broken.

Upon my arrival at the hospital, a pediatric orthopedic surgical physician was on call for orthopedic surgery. She determined that wrist and likely hip surgery would be necessary. She was about to prepare me for the wrist surgery. While on the operating room table, I was bumped in favor of a more serious emergency. Of course I didn't know that at the time, but in my lifetime I had never put a patient on the surgical table prepared for surgery, then took them off in favor of someone else. So I got angry. My excuse was the narcotic, although my wife continues to tell everyone it was just my personality because I wasn't in control. Whatever the case, the decision worked out for the best because the next day I got a specialist hand-surgeon who did a marvelous job, piecing me together with a metal plate and 11 screws. It took them some time to decide whether to operate on the hip, and eventually they decided it would heal best on its own without surgery. They made the correct decision. So I celebrated our son's birthday that year while sedated in the hospital. I went home after two weeks with a cast and a specialized walker and wheel chair. Getting me in the house was a challenge since I couldn't negotiate the steps. Once inside, I didn't go out for weeks. It wasn't fun but it was good to be alive. Our oldest son came to visit a few weeks later. The two 'boys', big as they were, managed to get me outside and push me down the driveway and down Rocky Road for an outing in my wheelchair. It was good to get outside. They pushed for quite awhile. I think we all forgot that pushing me back up the hill at 10,000 feet was going to be a struggle, clearly not for me but for them. It gave me some pleasure, though, to watch them struggle and fight for air as I sat in the chair. I admired their determination when there wasn't much choice.

When friends came to visit or called, I
frequently heard: "What were you doing on the
roof? Jews don't go on roofs". I related the story
to my brother, who in his own way with his dry
sense of humor said, "What do you mean Jews
don't go on roofs? Haven't you ever heard of
'Fiddler on the roof'"? I smiled and felt validated.

The CT scanner at the Telluride Medical Center
has served the community and my family well.
After living in town for over a year, I had been
asked by the Medical Director of the Telluride
Medical Center to consider sitting on the Board
of Directors. The facility was in dire shape
physically and organizationally. It was in huge
debt to the Montrose Medical Center, which
administered the clinic and emergency
department. The emergency department was
supported by a mil levy tax assessed on real
estate in the Telluride Hospital District,
essentially all of San Miguel County. Most if not
all of the medical referrals from the clinic went to
Montrose Hospital at the time, so it was in their

financial interest to administer the Telluride facility. This facility was an old building owned by the Idarado Mining company. Board certified emergency medicine physicians had not yet been hired to the emergency staff. There was no private money being raised on a regular basis other than sporadic donations to support the Center. The Telluride Medical Center was the only medical facility in town and was an hour a half from the nearest larger hospital, and two and a half hour drive from the nearest trauma center with good cardiac and neurosurgical care. X-rays were inexplicably taking weeks to be read. I learned that it wasn't uncommon for someone to walk around town for weeks thinking they had a broken limb. Weeks later after the films were officially read in Montrose, the patient would receive a call that they could take their sling or cast off because the limb was not broken. This kind of treatment didn't foster confidence on the part of the locals. This is the way medicine was practiced when I was asked to join the Board of Directors.

There was a need for a Board of Directors because the mil levy generated substantial yet insufficient dollars from taxation to support emergency services. Community oversight of those tax dollars was necessary by law. Interestingly there had never been a physician on the Board of Directors. The Board members were all well -intentioned volunteers yet help was needed. So I volunteered to fill a vacated seat. During my first Board meeting when I saw the bottom line numbers of the business spread sheet, I asked a question that evidently had never been asked before. I was curious as to how the bottom line debt on the books to Montrose Hospital was going to be paid back. No one had been concerned about it and there was no clear answer forthcoming to a growing monthly debt applied to the Telluride side of the ledger. There was also no accounting for the value of the referrals to the hospital going in the other direction. No one was happy with the way the emergency part of the clinic was operating. In

general the place was not in good financial or
physical shape. The carpets were worn and old,
the walls and floors were in need of repair and
paint. Competent as the staff was there were
too many of them for the volume being seen.
Expenses to revenues generated were quite high.
Fortunately or unfortunately for some, I stirred
the pot, which clearly needed stirring.

About three months after joining the Board,
Montrose Hospital exercised their right to
withdraw from management of the clinic. The
contract expired, and they chose not to renew. It
was unexpected and put the facility at risk for
having to close its doors, despite skiing and head
injuries, broken bones, heart attacks, car
accidents, and just about everything else in the
way of emergencies. In addition they expected
compensation for the bottom line figure of
hundreds of thousands of dollars that clearly the
Clinic did not have. If bankruptcy were declared it
would leave the ski mountain and the town
without medical services. Backs against the wall,

medical communities feuding with each other, Montrose pulling out demanding money and leaving the facility with no internal administration, being on the Board suddenly became a full time challenging and uncompensated job. It was the epitome of community service but it was also a service that the community could not survive without.

The first order of business was to go through the hoops of applying for a mil levy increase on real estate taxes, which took time and some expertise to get the initiative on the local ballot before November. Then we had to find an administrator, and figure out what kind of staff changes needed to be made by year-end. The mil levy funds, if successful at the ballot, could only be applied to the emergency services and not to the clinic. So clinic staff had to be cut, a most unpleasant and unpopular task, but the volume of business wasn't there to support the number and expense of all the personnel, no matter how talented and popular some of them were. So cut we did, and the Board took the hit.

Getting people to vote to increase their own
taxes is always fraught with difficulty and usually
failure. After all, who wants to vote to tax
themselves for any thing? For whatever reasons I
became the public face of the campaign. I stood
at the local post office corner day after day
passing out flyers and talking to people about
why the mil levy was critical. Simply put, if
defeated there would be no emergency care in
Telluride. Lives would be in jeopardy and lost.
Who knew what would have happened to the ski
mountain, the lifeblood of the town? Everyone
showed up at the post office almost daily since
there was no mail delivery; people got their mail
through boxes at the post office. I began to be
recognized as the Med Center guy. I was on the
local radio, in the newspapers, and at public
election forums speaking out. My fellow Board
members said I had a silver tongue so I should
just keep doing what I was doing. I know I
stopped the same people more than once to

discuss the issues because it was easier for me to recognize everyone's dogs than the people themselves. When the final vote was tallied on Election Day the mil levy increase generated over a million dollars annually and won by 88% favorable vote. The Denver newspapers picked up on the fact that of all the statewide mil levy questions on ballots in all the localities in the State this one won by the biggest margin.

We began to hire board certified emergency physicians. A good group of concerned locals of whom I was a part started the Telluride Medical Capital Fund, which began as an annual wine dinner cooked by local chefs and a live auction. Over the next few years due to generosity of many locals, we were able to raise another million dollars for much needed equipment, including the CT scanner, digital radiology and emergency room equipment. This allowed us to send our x-ray films to Nighthawk in Australia where they were read instantly. Even Montrose Hospital didn't have digital radiology at the time.

We enlisted the help of a second homeowner cardiologist who volunteered his expertise and saturated the town and ski mountain with AED's (defibrillators) paid for with donated funds, establishing Telluride as a shining example of how a ski mountain should be equipped in case of cardiac emergency. As a result, lives were saved. It distressed me to read how cardiac deaths occurred in other ski areas because they lacked the installation of AED's, or head injuries were managed incorrectly because they did not have availability of a CT scanner like we did. In short, the facility turned around and became self-supporting, sustainable, and continues to this day to provide excellent medical care to locals and visitors alike.

So we got the CT scanner that has saved lives and made countless difficult diagnoses for townsfolk and visitors alike. I had no idea that I would someday be inside of it when it came to town. My daughter wound up inside of the machine as well. From the time she was a little kid we used to race on the mountain. If for no other reason than size and momentum I won for many years. But with determination she kept trying and trying. When she got older and became an excellent skier herself, she got closer and closer until one year when I was going as fast as I could and was on the edge she blew right by me. I lost control. I could hear her laughing with glee as she flew by. She missed me slamming on my brakes and flying off the side of the run into the trees in a great cloud of snow. When I gathered myself up from one of my worst face plants ever, put my gear back on and crawled up the side of the run through trees and boulders, I realized how lucky I was to still be alive. No more racing for me. She, on the other hand, progressed to Air Garden to tackle the jumps. On one occasion, competing with her brothers, she got so airborne that it was obvious to me while she was airborne that she was not going to land on her skis, which she didn't. Fortunately for her, a trip to the emergency room and inside the CT scanner revealed only a concussion and nothing more serious, although to this day she still says her wrist is not quite right.

Although not actively practicing medicine but still with an active medical license in Colorado, and the only Board Certified OB-GYN in the County, I wanted to be called by the ER doctors if they ever had a need in the emergency facility for my obstetrical services. I volunteered for any obstetrical emergencies at the Medical Center. I had no malpractice insurance since I was not practicing clinical medicine, but I figured that in an emergency and acting as a Good Samaritan I really didn't have too much to worry about. My presence for deliveries was only needed twice during the years.

The ER docs had no interest in ever delivering a baby at the Medical center at 8500 feet above sea level where oxygen was at a premium, with no blood banking or operating facilities, and with no neonatal care facilities. Mostly everyone in Telluride who was pregnant went to Montrose or

Durango. The problem was that the hospitals were both at least 1.5 hours or longer away, over mountain passes which at times were closed or treacherous due to rapidly changing weather conditions. On two occasions women came in to the facility in active labor and there was no time in either case to put them in an ambulance. I was called and in I came. The first was an easy term delivery with no problems.

The second one was a bit different. When I arrived at the facility and walked into the emergency department cubicle, I saw my son's math teacher sitting next to the woman on the gurney. For a moment I was perplexed why he would be there. Then I realized it was his wife on the gurney grunting away and calling for the 'eye doctor'. I quickly examined her and found with one push she was going to have a premature baby. The problem was that she was only about 26 weeks pregnant, 6 ½ months or so. The odds of a baby surviving at 8500 feet above sea level at 26 weeks were slim to none. Oxygen was at a premium for undeveloped lungs. We got the pregnant patient prepped and draped as fast as we could, I had her push once, and out came a 1 1/2 pound baby male that fit in the palm of my hand. A stat call went out to Grand Junction air flight neonatal team, but I had no idea how long it would take for them to get here by helicopter, land at the airport outside of town then motor in to the Medical Center. I thought back to my years as an intern under the Father of Neonatology at Pennsylvania Hospital, and went into rescue mode. We did have a small endotracheal tube. Although I hadn't intubated a baby this size in decades, it went remarkably well. IV fluids were out of the question since we had nothing to catheterize the umbilicus with or small enough to place in a vein in a premature baby this size. So it was going to be all about acid base and oxygenation, warmth, preventing body heat loss, digital x-rays to check for tube placement, and bagging the baby with oxygen since we didn't have a respirator. It was kind of amazing to watch the color of the baby change with the rate of bagging, correct tube placement, and a bit of luck. It went from amazing blue to amazing pink in seconds with just the slightest movement one way or the other of the endotracheal tube. His skin was so fragile and translucent that judging oxygenation was easy.

This went on for an hour and a half, the time it took for the flight crew to get assembled and get here. I was never happier to see a support crew. The neonatal nurses came with all the right equipment and took over immediately, squirted surfactant down the endotracheal tube to help expand the baby's lungs, put in fluid lines, got him set up on antibiotics and respirator settings, and flew him back to Grand Junction where we had already sent the Mom by ambulance so that she would be there when the baby arrived. The Dad went in the helicopter. To my amazement, five years later I was so happy to see a good outcome. This kid was walking down the street with his Dad, as normal as any five year old could be. Mother Nature is definitely strange and unpredictable at times, and truly amazing! If you have good protoplasm and genes, and good medical care, life is on your side.

For the first time in decades when Board terms expired there was now sufficient interest in the community such that for the three seats available, four people wanted to be on the Board. This necessitated a county wide public election for the Board seats and I was a candidate. It was all fun, local politics at its best, and a wholly unanticipated experience for me. I was now an elected official.

Before I left for Africa I established a professional web site, essentially an electronic business card that highlighted key aspects of my past medical career. The major areas of my past experience that I emphasized were practice management, medical legal consulting, pharmaceutical and medical device research, and medical industry consulting. I felt I had knowledge and expertise I wanted to share, but on my own terms. I had an 800 number listed on the web site, my curriculum vitae, a picture and biographical background, and an email contact. Somehow people who were interested in an OB-GYN consultant found my website. I clearly had a disclaimer on the site that I was not looking to dispense medical advice over the Internet to individual patients, something I considered unethical without the ability to examine the patient. I was grateful that the business took off faster than what I had imagined it would.

My business generated some interesting twists. I received a call from a 'Young and Restless' TV soap opera producer to consult on a story line about keeping a pregnant pre-eclamptic woman in a coma for a while. I consulted with a Wall Street firm interested in understanding the potential of a new medical device being brought to market. I did work for a Pharmaceutical company on a new hormone trial on which they were about to embark. I did some practice management consultations, helping other physicians with difficult business decisions they needed to make. But by far the largest part of my new business was the medical legal expert witness consulting. Interestingly, though all the medical legal work I did while still practicing medicine was for defense of physicians, once I accepted one case for the plaintiff, the defense work disappeared. It was as if I had become a traitor now that I was willing to testify on behalf of patients who had indeed been maligned. So it was plaintiff's attorneys that found me, often either by word of mouth or by repeat business. I enjoyed the work. I could spend the morning skiing, come home to a nice warm mountain retreat, and spend part of the afternoon on the phone either discussing new cases with inquiring attorneys, or reading through medical charts that had been sent for me to review and offer opinions. I would write opinion letters, accept or reject cases that came my way depending on my sense and established written best practice standards of the American College of OB GYN. I would either arrange for my depositions to occur in the town of Telluride, or I would travel as necessary, both for depositions and trials. I had no payroll, no staff, no office problems, and no mutinous partners to deal with. The new professional role I had created suited me just fine.

Nothing in life, however, remains the same for too long. My wife had devoted most of her adult life continuing her education while being the primary care giver for our family. I was clearly involved in raising our family since other than medicine my family life was my primary interest. I didn't play cards, hit the bars at night, golf, or find other things to do that kept me away from home. When I wasn't working, I was always involved with family life by choice. But I worked a lot, and that kept me on the go away from home a lot, which was just the way life was for me. My wife was clearly the major source of a steady home life, homemaker, bread maker, Mom, and daily constancy for the kids. Before we left Arizona, she completed her Bachelor's degree in studio arts, years earlier having left her

first career as a medical laboratory technician.
She produced art, she taught art in the school
districts, she instructed the kids in art, and she
got involved with the local art therapy
community, her true love. Then it was no
surprise that when we were in Colorado, she
decided to pursue advanced education and
received her Master's degree in Art Therapy and
Counseling. During the educational process, she
worked with various local internships in Colorado
to complete counseling requirements. When she
graduated, she then decided to seek employment
in the field, and found a permanent position with
the State of California, which required another
move for us. By this time in our life, we were
open to change and looked at it both as a
challenge and a new experience for us. My
consulting business was portable, so off to
California we went for the next four years of our
life. Our kids were all gone from home, and we
were free to relocate. Once again friends said to
us: " How can you leave Telluride for California?"
particularly at a time when everyone travelling
on the interstate was leaving California for

Colorado. We were once again in touch with our nomadic genes, as we called them, and didn't mind swimming upstream away from what everyone else was doing. There was no longer a fear of the unknown. We embraced change, and the excitement it brings.

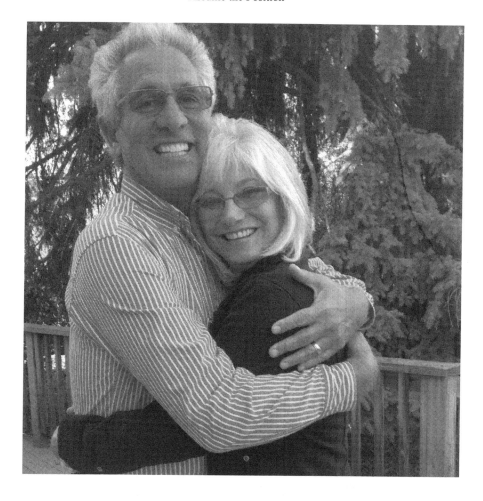

Although actively licensed in medicine, I became subject to more criticism from the witness stand, and it just wasn't where I wanted to be. The case at hand needed to be the focus, not me. I too needed a change of direction. And I needed to be supportive of my wife's desires and aspirations for her new career.

As a licensed physician, there are many paths to explore and many directions in which one can turn if so inclined. Fear is the only reason not to do so. An MD degree is a valuable and portable degree, especially if one is open to new and challenging things. I eventually found employment as a medical director for a Philadelphia based company with a new office located in California and went back to work. I had skiing out of my system, and enjoyed the opportunity to continue to use my medical knowledge on a daily basis. I was surprised how much information about general medicine was still in my head. As I tell people, I used to be a physician before I was an obstetrician, and I still am a physician. It was nice to be working for someone else, especially a large corporation owned by someone else, and watch others deal with the business headaches. I didn't always agree with their business decisions, but I enjoyed the work I was doing, found it quite easy, and no one was asking me for my opinions on how to run the business anyhow. That wasn't my role anymore. There were no malpractice issues about which to worry. Admittedly, when I started, I was a bit apprehensive having been out of active practice for a while. I needed to learn new computer skills, and dealing with medical issues outside of Obstetrics and Gynecology, but it didn't take me long to get up to snuff. They provided all the training necessary to do the job. So it turned out to be a good fit for them and for me.

After retiring from active practice, I incorrectly assumed that my acquired sleep disorder would at some time disappear. Now that years have gone by, there seems little hope that will ever happen. Years of up and down at all hours of the night, the necessity to be instantly awake when called upon to make at times life and death decisions, the need to give orders over the phone to the nursing staff and to direct patients what to do and when to do it, driving back and forth in the middle of the night, performing surgery and/or deliveries have all left me with a pattern of sleep that is hard to change. I have tried just about everything, including medications, and now simply just deal with myself as I am. I can fall asleep at the drop of a hat, but rarely can I stay asleep for more than 3-4 hours straight, after which I wrestle with my covers and myself the rest of the night. I wander around the house in the middle of the night when I am unable to fall back asleep, and eventually distract myself and my thoughts sufficiently that I can usually fall asleep again, but for only short intervals for the rest of the night. If one were to add up the hours, I suppose it is enough sleep, at least for me, but never what I feel is truly restful.

As I inevitably age, as we all do, we tend to find ourselves sitting on the exam table in front of other physicians. Most of my life I was comfortable seeing a physician every day by just looking in the mirror and making a quick assessment. But that isn't always going to work.

So now I have turned myself over to others and just bite the bullet like everyone else in the world. I have many observations about the state of medicine now, most of which I won't share. I simply will discuss two of them.

Obamacare. What an interesting word. I assume the term is at least partially patterned after Medicare, a program in which I now participate because the calendar tells me I am eligible. But take Obama out of Obamacare and substitute 'Medi' again, and we are back to where we should be. Why reinvent the wheel? I am intimately familiar with the medical side of Medicare, since most of the work I did as a medical director involved hospitals and Medicare patients. I find it most interesting that the conservative side of the political isle denigrates government medicine and government intervention in medicine. I believe current statistics will show that almost 18% of the Federal budget is Medicare dollars, a rather astounding figure of billions of dollars. The simple fact is that the system works. Even those who denigrate Obamacare on TV, in Congress, and wherever they have the chance to pontificate still belong to Medicare and utilize it. Why? Because overall it is a good system, it works, it keeps people healthy, and it keeps them from financial disaster when illness strikes, as it will for the elderly. It pays hospitals and providers. It just works! Sure, it has problems, but so does everything that chews up a large part of the federal budget. After all, isn't paying several thousand dollars for a toilet seat an important part of the Defense budget? Come on folks, let's get real. Take the greed and selfishness out of medicine where it has no place. Keep fixing the problems, keep auditing hospitals and doctors offices, keep returning money to the federal government when the audits produce millions of dollars of overpayments and expose fraud. Isn't that what elected officials are paid to do? Including the President, whomever he or she may be. Manage the government and exhibit fiscal responsibility. But don't scuttle programs that work for everyone, and which keep us healthy and out of financial ruin. Which brings me back to Obamacare. The system we have is what we have because of some sort of compromise forced upon us by the vocal minority and the Democrats who couldn't stand up for what they knew was right. If any system doesn't work properly, just fix it and make it better. Kind of like what we do with disease systems in medicine. The easier and wiser path would have been to just extend Medicare to people under the age of 65. How many millions were wasted in initiating and keeping a new program up and going? The system was already in place, it already works, and even though Republicans hate government intruding into our lives, better to be alive and solvent than poor before one dies. Government running medicine, they say. Horror upon horrors! It will never work. Just like Medicare and the VA don't work, yet keep millions of us alive and functioning well as vital parts of society while we age long beyond what anyone thought possible just decades ago. Government managed medicine – I am all for it. And just think how much money will be saved as we watch the private medical insurance business slowly drift off into the sunset where it belongs! Billions of dollars of profit in the insurance industry returned to investors. Why should there be profit in sickness and the medical insurance industry? Do we really want to profit from other people's misfortunes? Doctors and hospitals can be well paid without the private insurance sector. Don't get rid of government medicine, expand it, fix it, audit it, and keep it healthy. How many Republicans over the age of 65 do you hear complaining about Medicare? None, you say! Why not? Because they are happy with it, like everyone else; they just don't have the courage and honesty to tell you so.

My second pet peeve is computerized medicine. I grew up in the era before computers. I actually graduated from college without having ever used one, if one can still imagine that. But I embrace them fully, love them as much as the next guy, and can't imagine life without them. Computers and technology have changed medicine forever, and mostly for the better. But we still have a way to go. When I go into a doctor's office now, usually before the physician even comes into the room, as I sit in my gown on the exam table and assume my new position in life, I usually sit and stare at the computer which the nurse has turned on awaiting the arrival of the doctor, or watch as the doctor comes into the room carrying her laptop. If only the computer could talk then I wouldn't even need the physician and man and machine could get down to the exam! But we aren't quite there yet! He or she then arrives, sits down and begins talking, and typing. In other words, something has come between the physician and the patient. It used to be only a stethoscope. I appreciate fully how this has happened, why, and understand the utility of efficient electronic medical records. Heck, I would even embrace the implantation of a small silicone chip under the skin of a newborn baby at birth that would forever allow that individual to carry his or her medical records with him everywhere he goes, forever. It would have far more utility than a circumcision. Simply get scanned at the beginning or end of every medical encounter, whether conscious by consent or without consent when unconscious, extracting old information and entering new as necessary. Bingo! There is your medical history on the computer in front of your health care provider, who may need it to save your life at that very instant. It is done at the grocery store with bar codes and a scanner. I just miss the way a physician and patient interact without a machine between them. However, I don't think that is in our future anymore. Life changes, as must we!

About the Author

"Are you aware you are making an entirely emotional decision by choosing to go into Obstetrics and Gynecology?" was the way my Professor of Internal Medicine responded to hearing I had not chosen his field, but rather Obstetrics and Gynecology, when he asked me which internship programs I would be applying to upon graduation from medical school.

At the time during my fourth year of medical school when I finally made this life long commitment, I can't say that I was aware of the emotional commitment I was making. To me it was a thoughtful decision that came after four years of higher education post high school, hours of studying, nights and weekends on call, examinations both written and oral, clinical rotations through all the specialties of medicine, endless lab sessions, and simply trying to figure out which parts of medicine interested me the

most, and the least.

I assessed myself as best I could. I needed intellectual stimulation. I needed an active and challenging life on a daily basis. I could not be sedentary. I was good with my hands and enjoyed surgery. I had received academic honors in both internal medicine and psychiatry yet I didn't want to choose either as a life long commitment. I loved the two elective rotations I had spent in Obstetrics and Gynecology.

Much of medicine I found depressing, not something I really had considered much before entering medical school. As important as many medical subspecialties are, for me I did not enjoy dealing with chronic diseases, nor did I enjoy the medical clinics that brought these patients in week after week with the same chronic complaints which necessitated pushing the same medications over and over again. I was not enamored with cancer and its ravages on the body and the person. It was painful for me to watch and care for dying patients.

I enjoyed the challenges of making a diagnosis based on my clinical acumen and diagnostic skills. I loved the variety of patients and problems that Obstetrics and Gynecology brought to the office. For me, the thrill of caring for otherwise healthy, young, hopeful women over a nine-month period of time to help them bring a healthy human being with all its potential into the world was exciting, then to send it off into the world as the picture of health with enormous god given potential. If the infant wound up having a difficult life, I didn't want it to be as a result of lack of good medicine when on my watch for nine months. I liked the fact that surgery was part of the specialty, such that with my hands, eyes, ears and thought processes I could use my talents and education to offer people immediate relief from problems amenable to surgical correction. I liked the fact that in one fashion or another almost every patient required some sort of counseling and reassurance before they left the office, even if they weren't aware of it. I enjoyed dealing with infertility issues and bringing happiness and joy to otherwise fearful patients who thought they would be childless. I often found myself in the midst of life cycle changing events of the women who presented to the office, and I appreciated the trust and responsibility placed in me to help them not only with their health but also achieving their goals in life. One's social status, age, financial status, heritage, race, religion or even values did not matter to me. I enjoyed the challenge of being totally non- discriminatory and accepting of whomever found their way into my office. I constantly strived never to preach, moralize, or make someone feel guilty or doubtful about the decisions they were making, regardless of how I might personally feel about their situation in life. This was often the biggest challenge of Obstetrics and Gynecology – to be non judgmental and accepting of everyone without hesitation or question, and simply to provide the patients with the best medical advice and care available under their particular unique circumstances with their reproductive, hormonal and emotional life often in the balance. It was indeed a yearly, monthly, daily, and often hourly challenge, day and night that required constant vigilance, perception, patience, and understanding.

As I came to realize, my Professor of Medicine was indeed correct. It was an emotional decision that I was making at the time. I just didn't know how much of one it was! Every single patient had emotions that needed to be assessed and discussed. Every single patient brought out emotions in me, none of which could be assessed and discussed. There wasn't time for me to deal with my own emotions while in clinical practice, because I was intimately involved with everyone else's.

One can imagine all the negatives one hears about going into the field of Obstetrics and Gynecology, often expressed by my medical colleagues themselves. I heard them all: "The hours are awful"; "The patients are needy"; " Your family life will be terrible"; " The smells can be overwhelming"; "You will always be exhausted and sleep deprived"; "Why would you want to deal with women all day long"; "It requires an inordinate amount of patience". These were but a few. But for me the positives far outweighed the negatives. The decision was made and my life was about to change forever – I hoped for the positive, because I was about to jump in 100%.

After 28 years in medicine, and 20 years in active clinical practice of Obstetrics and Gynecology in one of the largest group practices in Phoenix, Arizona, the medical vignettes I have recounted are all true; the fears I have tapped into, my own and those of many of my patients, are as they occurred; the trials and tribulations of my patients are recounted as accurately as possible with names deleted or changed. For many people, the life of an Obstetrician and Gynecologist is often the butt of many late night jokes at parties and on television. The mythology surrounding the specialty is extensive. I have tried to bring the patients and their stories to life. My personal experiences and thoughts in dealing with these patients, heretofore known only to me, have now seen daylight. Many readers will I am sure see their own fears and lives exposed; and many will be able to relate only in the sense that they are glad that none of these events and scenarios depicted have ever happened to them. Husbands, boyfriends, significant others will now know more about what goes on behind the closed doors of a world which many wonder about, and many choose not to enter. And perhaps for those considering the specialty in the future, this book will be an eye opener. Medicine in general requires dedication and love. It becomes our master. We cannot escape the fact that we are physicians until we hit the grave. But it is a fulfilling and all encompassing life from which one can learn a tremendous amount about the depth and breadth of the human species. It is a totally unselfish existence. At its core, it simply demands caring for other human beings.

39006391R00233

Made in the USA
Lexington, KY
03 February 2015